HATHA YOGA
Th e Complete Mind and Body Workout

JULIET PEGRUM

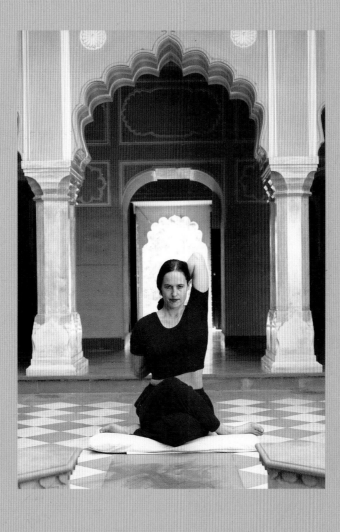

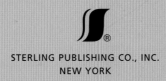

STERLING PUBLISHING CO., INC.
NEW YORK

Author's acknowledgments

To all my kind teachers who tirelessly share their wisdom and to all who seek happiness and freedom through the practices of yoga.

Juliet Pegrum can be contacted at: julietpegrum@mahamudrayoga.com

Published in 2003 by Sterling Publishing Co., Inc.
387 Park Avenue South, New York, NY 10016

First published in Great Britain in 2003 by
Cico Books
32 Great Sutton Street London EC1V 0NB

© 2003 Cico Books
Text © 2003 Juliet Pegrum

Distributed in Canada by Sterling Publishing
c/o Canadian Manda Group, One Atlantic Avenue
Suite 105, Toronto, Ontario, Canada M6K 3E7

Library of Congress Cataloging-in-Publication
Data available

10 9 8 7 6 5 4 3 2 1

ISBN 1-4027-0872-6

Project editor: Mary Lambert

Photography: Geoff Dann

Design: Jerry Goldie Graphic Design

Printed and bound in China

Contents

Introduction

Asato maa sat gamaya

Tamaso maa jyotir gamaya

Mrityor maa amritam gamaya

Om shanti, shanti, shanti.

Lead us from the unreal to the real

Lead us from darkness to the light

Lead us from the impermanent to the eternal

Om peace, peace, peace.

Yoga is more than a system of exercises—it is a sacred practice that leads to lasting peace and happiness. The ancient yogis declared that true happiness could not be found in the external world, by which we are repeatedly disillusioned. Rather, true freedom and bliss are found inside ourselves, in the silent place between words and thoughts that lies beyond the turmoil of life. Yoga provides the tools to connect to this transcendent peace and pure joy, which exists free of conditions.

Included in this chapter is an explanation of Hatha yoga; its philosophy; a description of how the subtle body energy flow works; the best diet to eat, and how food affects our body; plus a section on breathing and meditation.

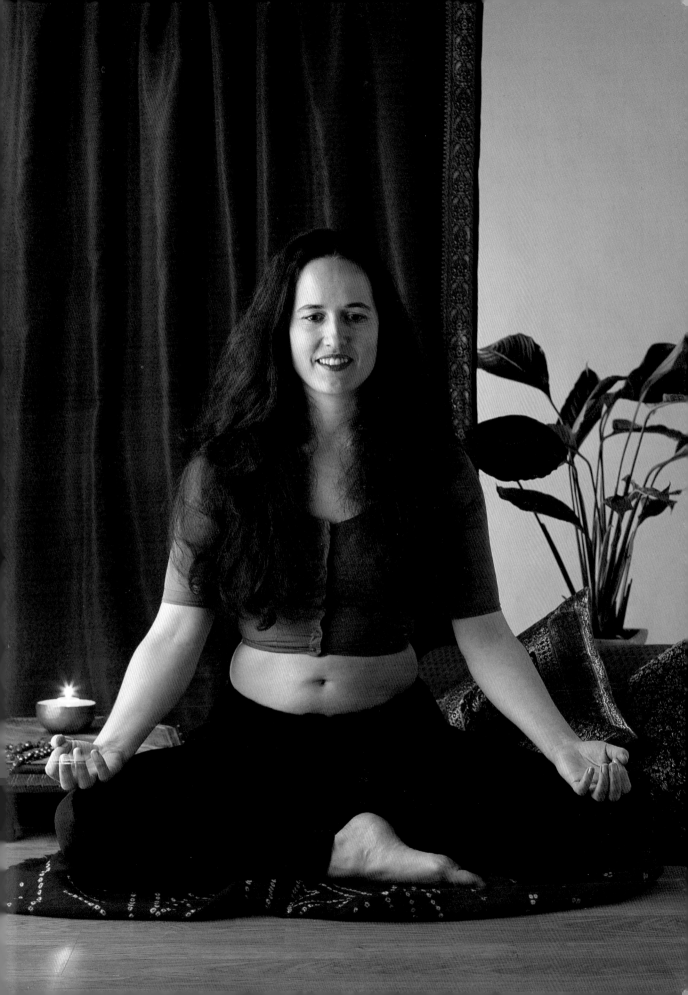

What is Hatha yoga?

The term "Hatha" literally means forceful or strong yoga. It refers to the different physical practices of yoga, which are asana, pranayama (breath control), and meditation (mental concentration). Hatha yoga was said to be a gift to mankind from the Hindu god Siva, as a method for attaining freedom from physical and mental suffering.

The physical poses of Hatha yoga have been described in ancient yoga texts of the *Hatha Yoga Pradipika*, the *Gheranda* and *Siva Samhitas*. The most popular yogi of the Hatha yoga tradition, who is revered as its inventor, is Gorakanath. He is believed to have come from Northern India and to have lived at some time between the 9th and 12th centuries. However, almost nothing is known of this historical figure as myth and legend has shrouded his whole life. Gorakanath is reputed to be the author of a text entitled *Hatha Yoga*, which is no longer in existence.

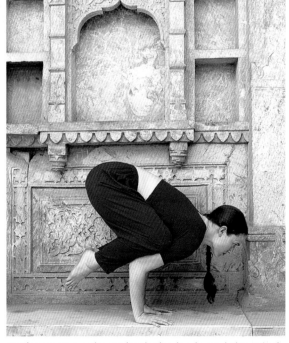

Hatha yoga works on both the body and the mind, encouraging a good flow of *prana*.

The ancients knew Hatha yoga as a therapeutic science. It is a precise system for purifying the body and mind that works on the physical and the subtle body layers. According to the Hatha yoga teachings, all the vital body functions are controlled by a subtle energy called *prana*. *Prana* is transmitted through thousands of energy channels called *nadis* that form a network in the body. It is believed that when energy is not flowing properly in a part of the body, toxins accumulate there, causing stiffness or pain. By regularly practicing Hatha yoga, the *prana* is moved positively through the body, clearing away all impurities to keep the body in good health.

HATHA YOGA POSES

Hatha yoga poses promote balance and harmony. They aid the circulatory, nervous, respiratory, hormonal, and digestive systems, and purify and detoxify the entire body. While the poses directly affect the body, when they are practiced in unison with the breath, they positively affect the mind. Yoga is a potent tool in counterbalancing the mental stress of everyday life, as it brings the mind into a state of calm.

Hatha yoga can be practiced by anyone, and you do not have to be very fit to begin yoga. It involves mastering a series of bodily postures, but it does not have to be a long, exhausting session. It is just as beneficial to practice Hatha yoga consistently for short periods, when your mind is fully absorbed in the exercise.

Yoga philosophy

The philosophy of yoga has been handed down through the yoga sutras (or sayings) written by Patanjali around 200–400 BC. Patanjali did not invent the system of yoga, but rather systemized the existing teachings, which are much older, into a concise eight-step path.

The eight-step path provides clear instructions on how to control the mind and sense organs to experience lasting bliss, and freedom from suffering. Patanjali is considered the father of yoga and his sutras form the essence of all the various types of yoga that flourish today.

THE EIGHT STEPS

A brief summary of the contents of the eight steps is provided here. For more in-depth information, it is advisable that you read the original sutras of Patanjali, which are widely available. The first two steps to yoga, the *yamas* (the restraints) and the *niyamas* (the observances) form the basic foundation of the practice. Together they comprise the ten virtuous actions. In our modern world, many people object to following a strict code of behavior, however, each of the eight steps is of equal importance, and to gain mastery of the mind, willpower has to be strengthened by using self-control. Also, to meditate well, you need a clear conscience, or the mind becomes restless.

THE EIGHT STEPS

Step 1 *Yamas*/Restraints
Ahimsa/non-violence is an attitude of not wishing to harm any living being, including oneself, in word, thought or action.
Satya/truthfulness is the ability to lead an honest and open life.
Asteya/non-stealing is not taking or using that which is not given.
Brahmacarya/conservation of energy is the moderation of the senses, avoiding excess or debauchery in sex, drugs or food.
Aparigraha/non-greed is abstention from greed, hoarding or hankering after the possessions of others.

Step 2 *Niyamas*/Observances
Saucha/purity is purity of mind and a natural disinterest in one's external appearance, while cultivating one's inner beauty.
Santosha/contentment is to be happy as we are, free from likes and dislikes.
Tapas/self-discipline is effort and the mental strength to accept hardship as part of the path.
Svadhyaya/study is the study of the scriptures.
Ishvarapranidhana/surrender is dedicating our activities and accomplishments to the benefit of others.

Step 3 *Asanas*/Poses
Yoga poses or asanas are defined in the yoga sutras as *sthirasukham*, meaning stable and agreeable. With regular practice of the poses (see Chapters 2–7), effort disappears, and is replaced by ease and steadiness of mind, in preparation for pranayama and meditation.

Step 4 *Pranayama*/Breath
The control and expansion of the life force through conscious breathing, which is outlined in Chapter 7.

Step 5 *Pratyahara*
The withdrawal of the senses from external stimuli (see pp.10–11).

Step 6 *Dharana*
Single-pointed concentration (see pp.10–11).

Step 7 *Dhyana*
Meditation (this is discussed further in Chapter 7).

Step 8 *Samadhi*
Unification of consciousness (see pp.10–11).

Types of yoga

Hatha yoga is a very powerful tool for toning the body and focusing the mind. The term "Hatha" is used collectively to name the traditional disciplines that are practiced to gain mastery of the body and mind, such as asana, pranayama, and meditation.

There are many types and schools of yoga that are available today, such as Iyengar yoga, Ashtanga yoga, and Sivananda yoga. All the various schools include the practices of hatha yoga, but the difference is in the style and approach. Some schools focus more on movement and the continuous flow from one posture to the next, while others emphasize correct alignment and holding each pose for a longer time.

A yoga class can be energetic and physically demanding, or more meditative and restorative, depending on the poses practiced, the speed at which they are performed, and the length of time for which the poses are held. It is interesting to note that one Indian Master, Sri Krishnamacharya, instigated three schools of yoga, each with a very different emphasis on how it is performed. He is considered to be the grandfather of Ashtanga yoga, Iyengar yoga, and Viniyoga.

"There are many paths leading to the same goal" is a popular Indian saying. Each individual's constitution is unique and the various forms of yoga that are available complement these differences. When you are looking for a yoga class, it is advisable to try out a few different styles until you find the one that suits you. Just to give you an idea where you can start looking, here is a brief outline of the practices of a few of the most popular schools of yoga.

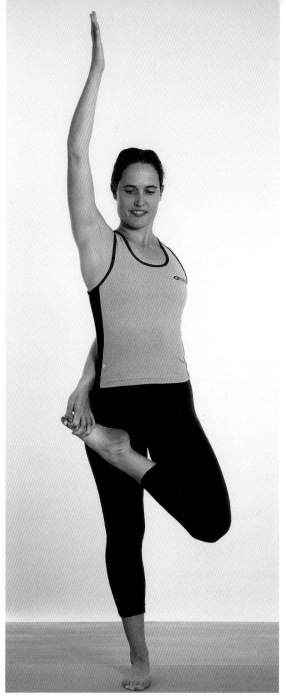

This half-bound lotus stretch is one of the standing poses of the Ashtanga yoga school.

ASHTANGA

Shri Pattabhi Jois in Mysore, South India, developed Ashtanga yoga, which is sometimes called "power yoga." Ashtanga yoga is a dynamic, flowing sequence of set poses that links the movements with the breath. It quickly builds stamina and increases the body's flexibility, but for beginners to yoga, it can be a physically demanding practice.

BIKRAM

Started by Bikram Choudry in California, Bikram yoga has a set sequence of twenty-six poses plus two breathing exercises. The classes tend to be sweaty, as they are held in a room heated to about 85°F/30°C. This extreme heat aids flexibility and suppleness. Each pose is repeated twice and held for at least 10 seconds. The practice is rigorous and makes a really good workout.

INTEGRAL

Swami Satchidanada, a student of Swami Sivananda, founded Integral Yoga in the U.S. It is a gentle style of yoga that integrates a variety of techniques, including asana, pranayama, chanting, and meditation. It encourages students to work within their own limits, and to develop awareness throughout the practice.

IYENGAR

B. K. S. Iyengar, who lives in Pune, India, started Iyengar yoga. It is the most popular form of yoga practiced in the West. He stresses correct body alignment and an understanding of how it is structured. He was also the great innovator of yoga props, such as blocks and belts, making asana practice accessible to all. The classes are detail-oriented and informative.

KUNDALINI

Kundalini yoga was founded by Sikh Yogi Bhajan. Kundalini is an ancient and esoteric practice designed to awaken the vital energy that lies dormant at the base of the spine. The practice emphasizes chanting and breathing, along with asana, to stir the vital energy within. The primary focus of this yoga is on the breath.

SIVANANDA

Vishnu Devananda, a disciple of Swami Sivananda, started the Sivananda style of yoga. The yoga practice incorporates asana, breathing, and deep relaxation. The classes are relaxed and gentle.

VINIYOGA

The son of Sri Krisnamacharya, T. K. V. Desikarchar, teaches Viniyoga in Madras, South India. His style of Hatha yoga focuses on the needs of the individual and includes asana, chanting, pranayama, and meditation. The pace is gentle, with awareness on the breath—postures are seen as an expression of the breath. All the postures are modified to suit the student.

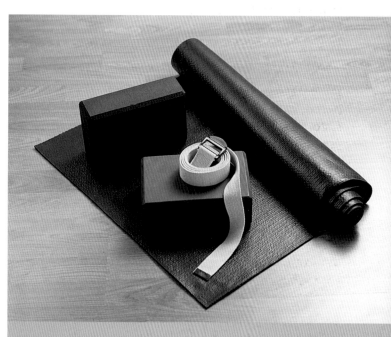

YOGA EQUIPMENT

B. K. S. Iyengar was responsible for first introducing yoga equipment for use by beginners to yoga. Most classes today now incorporate them. The sticky mat is used to lie or stand on during the poses. The belts help a beginner stretch into a pose more easily, and the blocks are used to support the body, or to help a beginner achieve a strenuous pose more easily.

Energy channels

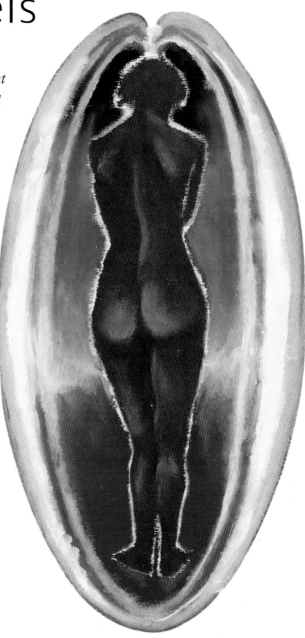

We think of our physical body as one entity, but according to the teachings of yoga, the physical body is made up of five layers or sheaths. Each layer leads from the physical to the more subtle or ethereal layers of existence.

The purpose of yoga practice is to reconnect to the most subtle, underlying nature of being. The various yoga practices, such as asana, pranayama, and meditation work directly with these different layers.

THE FIVE LAYERS

The gross physical body, *Annamaya kosha*, is toned and strengthened through asana practice. The second layer, *Pranamaya kosha*, refers to the energetic body. The energetic body animates the physical body and comprises the network of subtle energy channels called *nadis*, along which *prana* or energy flow. Pranayama or the breath works to tone and remove any obstacles that exist in the energetic body.

The third layer, the *Manomaya kosha*, or mental body, encompasses the conscious, sub-conscious and instinctive aspects of the mind. When you are withdrawing your senses in preparation for meditation, you work with this body. The fourth layer, the wisdom body or *Vijnanamaya kosha*, is the seat of intuition, greater awareness, understanding, and discrimination. The practice of one-pointed concentration connects with the wisdom body. The fifth and the most subtle layer, the *Anandamaya kosha*, or bliss body, is beyond the mental and physical aspects of the body and is experienced as pure joy and unconditional love, which is only reached through deep meditation practice.

The body is made up of five layers, according to yoga teachings. Here the first three layers are shown.

As the yoga practices work on both the gross and the subtle layers of the body, it is useful to have an understanding of the subtle energetic body as outlined in the yoga scriptures. Energy flows through the body along a vast network of channels—the *nadis*. There are said to be 72,000 *nadis* in the body that conduct energy through it. Some people believe that the channels relate to the nervous system, and the sympathetic and the parasympathetic nerves.

THE AIM OF HATHA YOGA

The word Hatha comprises "ha" meaning sun and "tha" meaning moon. This refers to two major energy channels (*nadis*) that extend from the base of the spine up to the *ajna* chakra located in the center of the forehead.

In the practice of yoga, three of the *nadis* are of primary importance: the *Sushumna nadi*, the *Pingala nadi*, the sun channel and the *Ida nadi*, the moon channel. *Sushumna*, the most important *nadi*, flows from the base of the spine to the crown of the head in line with the spinal column. On the right of the *Sushumna nadi*, running up as far as the *ajna* chakra is "ha," the sun channel. The sun channel is the active male principal within the body. The male energy activates the physical body and governs the right side, transmitting data from the left side of the brain, the rational hemisphere. On the left of the *Sushumna nadi*, running up to the *ajna* chakra is "tha," the moon channel.

The moon channel is the female principle, which transmits consciousness to every part of the body and controls the left side, sending messages from the right side of the brain, the artistic and creative hemisphere. Hatha yoga aims to balance the two forces in the body—the male and female energies. The practice helps to ensure that the alternating functions of the two *nadis* are in harmony for the benefit of the whole physical and mental system. That is why most of the yoga exercises stretch and strengthen both sides of the body equally.

In addition to harmonizing the left and right sides and all the bodily activities, yoga practice, by unifying the male and female aspects, aims to awaken the subtle energy of creation itself. This energy, referred to as *kundalini*, lies dormant at the base of the spine just above the *muladhara* chakra. When awakened, *kundalini* enters the central channel and rises up to the crown of the head, cutting all bonds to the relative plane of existence—it leads to *samadhi*, the blissful, transcendent state of being.

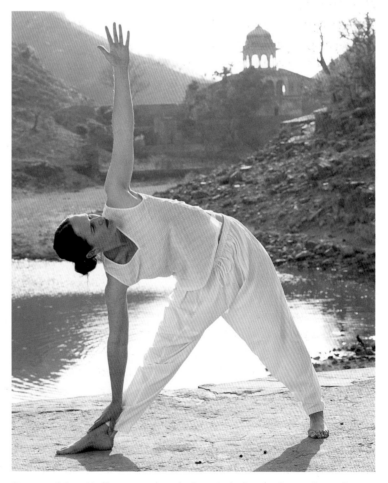

By practicing Hatha yoga regularly, you balance the male and female energies that exist in your body.

The chakras

THE SEVEN BODY CHAKRAS

At certain points along the *sushumna* or vertebral column, the nadis come together and form nerve plexuses or centers of energy called chakras. A chakra literally translates as spinning wheel, because at these locations energy gathers and pulsates at a certain vibration, causing a swirling motion. There are many chakras located over the body, but there are seven main ones that are essential to yoga and other spiritual practices.

The five lowest chakras are connected to the five elements or constituents of creation: earth, water, fire, air, and ether. Each element is considered to be condensed energy, vibrating at a different frequency. At the bottom of the spectrum, and connected to the first chakra, is the element earth, which has the lowest vibration and the densest structure. The chakra system follows a similar model to the five bodies, moving from the most solid element, earth, to the most ephemeral, ether or space. The two highest chakras move beyond the physical and connect to the spiritual realm.

Each of the elements connects to one of the five senses, through which we experience the physical world.

Yoga aims at purifying, cleansing and attuning the chakras to a higher frequency in preparation for the awakening of *kundalini*. It is possible to direct *prana* or energy to a chakra by fixing your attention and sending the breath to it, causing *prana* to follow. This is the secret behind pranic- or self-healing. Each chakra of the five lower chakras has a bija or seed syllable or corresponding sound associated with it. Chanting the seed mantra also activates the chakra.

1 *Muladhara*—foundation center. This chakra is located at the base of the body in the perineal floor, between the anus and the sexual organs, and governs the adrenal glands and lower pelvic area. It is associated with the earth element, which is connected to our sense of smell. The bija mantra for this chakra is "LAM." This center is connected to basic survival and physical stability, and is related to money, community and family.

2 *Svadisthana*—creative center. This chakra is located about two inches above the first, around the area of the prostate gland or uterus and is associated with these organs, plus the kidneys, bladder and intestines. It corresponds to the water element and the sense of taste. The bija mantra for this chakra is "VAM." It represents our creative side, procreation, and is our sexual and vital energy center.

3 *Manipura*—transformation center. This chakra is located around the navel area, and is connected to the digestive system, the spleen and liver. It is associated with the fire element, and the corresponding sense is sight. Like fire, the digestive system transforms all that it is fed into energy. The bija mantra for this chakra is "RAM." This chakra is connected to our willpower and the sense of ourselves or self-image.

4 *Anahata*—compassion center. This chakra is located at the center of the chest where the heart is. It governs the lungs, heart, arms, and hands. It is connected to the air element and the sense of touch, indicated by our ability to reach out and hug others. The bija mantra is "YAM." It is said that through this chakra we connect to humanity, and it reflects our ability to give or receive love.

5 *Vishuddhi*—communication center. This chakra is located in the throat, close to the larynx. It is connected to the tonsils, vocal cords, thyroid and

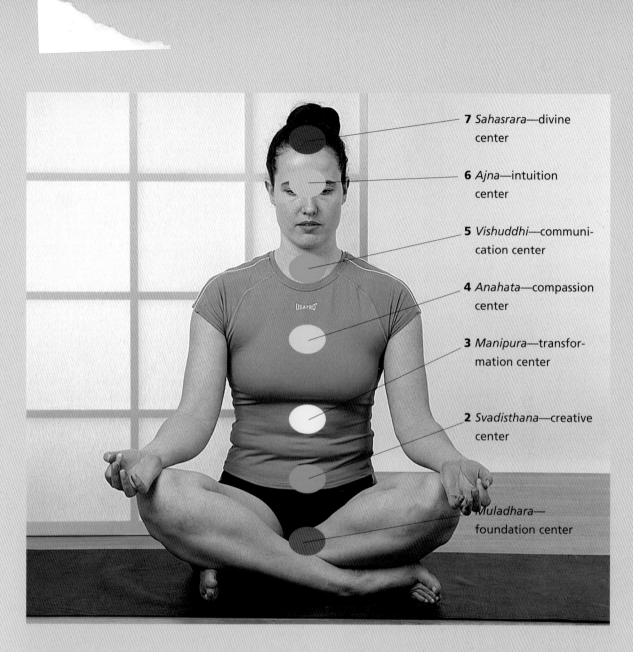

7 *Sahasrara*—divine center

6 *Ajna*—intuition center

5 *Vishuddhi*—communication center

4 *Anahata*—compassion center

3 *Manipura*—transformation center

2 *Svadisthana*—creative center

Muladhara—foundation center

parathyroid glands. Space or ether is the associated element and hearing is the sense. The bija mantra is "HAM." This chakra governs our ability to communicate, to listen, and to be heard.

6 *Ajna*—intuition center. This chakra is the first center that moves beyond the physical and the five elements and is located at the top of the spinal column at the area between the eyebrows. It is connected to the pituitary and pineal glands. This is the area where the *Sushumna, Ida*, and *Pingala nadis* all meet. This center is connected to the sixth sense, intuition or the third eye and the metaphysical world. Like the god Mercury, the *ajna* chakra is the mediator or intermediate step between the physical and the spiritual levels of existence. It is connected to mercy, and the ability to forgive both others and ourselves.

7 *Sahasrara*—divine center. This chakra is located at the crown of the head and is said to be beyond both mind and matter. It is connected to the pineal gland and the brain, and represents pure consciousness before it is fragmented by thought and scattered by the five senses. When pure energy or *kundalini* is unbound and rises up to the *sahasrara* chakra, illumination occurs, like switching on a light bulb, and the darkness of misconceptions, and ignorance, are removed. It is connected to a love of life, and kindness and compassion toward others.

Mudras

The word "mudra" is derived from an Assyrian word meaning imprint or seal. Mudras are subtle movements, gestures, or physical expressions that embody a spiritual meaning. They represent a symbolic language that transmits esoteric ideas.

The most well known mudras are made with the hands, although there are also head and postural mudras. Postural mudras combine a pose with a particular type of breath. It is said that a yoga asana, when it has been perfected, becomes a mudra.

THE MEANING OF MUDRAS

Hand signs occur in every culture throughout the world, and are literally thoughts in form. Studies have shown that hand gestures emanate from a primitive area of the brain—the right side close to the brain stem. A gesture will spring forth—like waving "hello"—before a verbal thought, which is located in the left brain and linked to rational activity, enters the mind. Therefore, mudras short-circuit the intellect and communicate directly to the right brain, where unconscious and instinctive responses are stored, helping to reconfigure the mind at a much deeper level. Research on mudras has shown that they imprint a similar frame of mind or neural firings in the brain of both the practitioner and also the observer.

PRACTICING THE MUDRAS

■ Traditionally, mudras were considered to be a higher spiritual practice and they were only introduced after an aspirant was accomplished in both asana and pranayama. They set up different energy currents in the body, redirecting energy or *prana* that would normally be dissipated, back into the body, which then alters perception or mood.

■ Mudras help to deepen concentration by maintaining awareness on a fixed point, such as the *jnana* mudra used in meditation. The *jnana* mudra means wisdom or the gesture of intuitive knowledge. It is a psycho-neural finger lock where the index finger touches the root of the thumb. The index finger represents individual consciousness and the thumb symbolizes supreme consciousness. The mudra therefore represents the unity of consciousness experienced in *samadhi*.

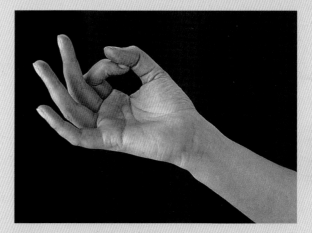

Jnana mudra
Wisdom gesture
Folding the index finger to touch the root of the thumb forms *Jnana* mudra. It can also be performed with the tips of the thumb and index finger touching. *Jnana* mudra is used during meditation and symbolizes the surrender of the individual to the divine consciousness.

Meru mudra
Offering gesture

This is a complicated mudra in which the palms are open and the little fingers are crossed, with the right thumb touching the tip of the left little finger, and the left thumb touching the right. The ring fingers are extended upward with the knuckles touching. The middle fingers are crossed with the right index finger wrapped around the left middle finger and the left wrapped around the right. The *meru* mudra is used as an offering gesture, giving the entire universe. The extended ring fingers represent Mount Meru, the mythical golden mountain that serves as the abode of all the deities.

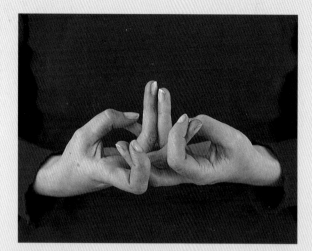

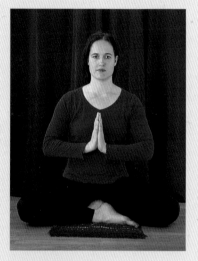

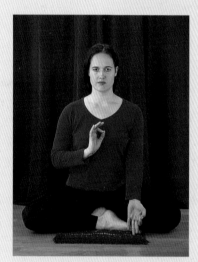

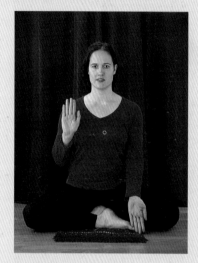

Anjali mudra
Adoration gesture

Placing the palms of your hands together at your heart brings the left and the right sides of the brain, or male and female energies, into harmony. In India, the *anjali* mudra is used as a greeting, and as a reverent gesture to the divine within each person.

Vitarka mudra
Instruction gesture

First adopt *jnana* mudra with both hands together and then place your right hand in front of your heart, while resting your left hand on your left knee to form *Vitarka* mudra. Lord Buddha made this mudra after his first sermon to symbolize the exchange of knowledge between teacher and student.

Abhaya mudra
Fearless gesture

Raise the right hand with your palm facing forward to the level of your shoulder, and place your left hand down on your left knee with the fingers pointing toward the earth. *Abhaya* mudra is a very open gesture that transmits a feeling of safety and a signal to approach. Holding the left palm open, with the fingers down, symbolizes forgiveness.

Diet and cleansing

*Diet plays an important role in our day-to-day health and wellbeing.
Eastern thinking is that there are two main sources of energy that sustain
our bodies: the air that we breathe and the food that we eat.*

According to the yogic scriptures, food can be divided into three different types or energy, *sattva*, *rajas*, and *tamas*. The qualities of *sattva* are tranquility, clarity, and cohesion; of *rajas* restlessness, activity, and passion, and of *tamas*, dullness and lethargy. These energies are taken into our system through all the different foods that we eat.

Natural, fresh foods that are not spicy in any way are considered *sattvic*. These include fruits, nuts, yogurts, vegetables, cooked grains, and cereal. Foods that are spicy, pungent, and sour are *rajasic*. These include garlic, onions, chilis, meat, fish, and alcohol—all of these foods cause restlessness and desire in the mind. All foods that are old, processed, cold, and over-cooked are *tamasic*, causing laziness and a feeling of inertia.

The three main causes of disease are stress, toxins, and bad eating habits. The way in which we eat affects the quality of the food. Digestion begins in the mouth, so food that is not chewed sufficiently ferments in the stomach and produces toxicity in the system.

It is never advisable to eat when you are upset, angry, or in a hurry as you will not chew your food properly.

A BALANCED DIET

A healthy diet is one that contains nutritious, easily digestible food. A good diet should help to maintain clarity and tranquility of mind, and will not stiffen the body. Through eating a proper diet, the body is cleansed, toxins are eliminated, and the vitamins and minerals that are required are easily absorbed. The aim of yoga is to lead a simple, healthy and natural life. So fresh, *sattvic* foods are the staple diet of a yogi. Moderation is also the paradigm of yoga—it is better to eat small regular meals than to eat too much in one sitting, or to fast excessively.

As a commitment to protect all sentient life, the first restraint of yoga philosophy is non-killing of animals. Therefore, yogis tend to adopt a

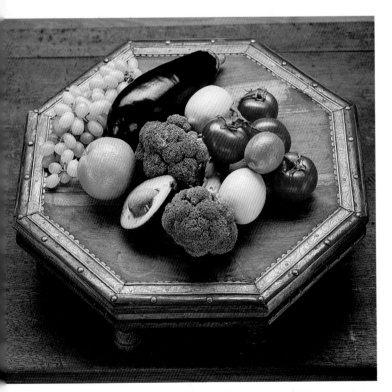

Fresh, sattvic foods, such as fruit and vegetables, are the staple diet of a yogi, and should form a major part of your daily diet if you practice yoga.

CLEANSING

Fasting occasionally is a good way to cleanse and purify your system. It is recommended to fast for a day once or twice a month, or for a weekend several times a year. A total fast consists of only drinking water, while for a lighter fast, fresh juices can be taken.

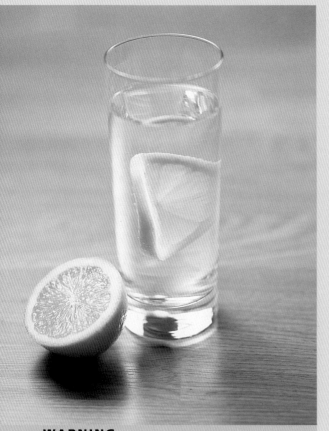

WARNING
Do not attempt to fast if you are pregnant or suffering from anemia.

■ Fasting gives your digestive system a rest, and allows toxins that have accumulated in your body to be eliminated. While fasting, it is important to drink lots of water to flush out your system. It is better to fast in a natural environment where there is an abundance of fresh air. Try to remain as quiet and relaxed as much as you can during a fast, and do not attempt anything strenuous. You may experience some side effects, such as headaches and nausea, which are a natural part of the elimination process. So if you suffer from these, just drink some more fluids.

■ To break the fast, it is important to take something light, such as soup or steamed vegetables, on the first day and then as your body adapts, you can move on to more complex meals.

■ A daily method of cleansing is to drink a glass of squeezed lemon juice and warm water in the morning, when you first get up, and then wait for at least 30 minutes before eating any other food or drink.

vegetarian diet. However, rather than embarking on a new dietary regime, you will find the desire to overeat, or eat junk food, will naturally disappear as your body and mind are purified through the practice of asana and pranayama.

Traditionally, before eating a meal it is good to reflect on where the food has come from, and how the energy from the food can be used most nobly. Also it is good to give thanks to the abundant earth by offering up a special prayer.

Breathing

Breath control is one of the most important aspects in the path of yoga. Pranayama, which is the control and expansion of vitality using the breath, is an advanced yoga practice.

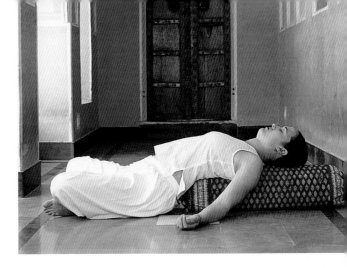

Ujjayi breathing is best practiced while lying on the floor with a bolster supporting your spine and ribs.

Pranayama is not traditionally taught to people doing yoga until mastery of the body has been attained through the practice of asanas. An in-depth explanation of pranayama, along with some simple preparatory exercises, are outlined on pages 110–112.

However, correct breathing is integral to the yoga postures and there are a few general guidelines to follow while you are practicing. You always need to breathe through your nose, as this automatically regulates the flow of air into your lungs. The nostrils act as a natural filter, removing dust and germs from the air. The nasal passages warm the air to the perfect temperature for absorption by the lungs, without causing damage to the delicate organs. When your sinuses are not used effectively they become congested and blocked. So, consciously breathing through the nose during practice helps to keep them clear. In certain strenuous postures, your breathing may become labored, and there can be a tendency to breathe through the mouth, in which case slow down and resume nostril breathing.

EVEN BREATHING
When breathing, try to make your inhalation the same length as your exhalation. Keep your breaths in and out long, deep, and rhythmic like the sound of waves against the shore. The breath should never be retained for long periods while practicing asanas. When you apply too much effort and concentration during a pose, there is an inclination to hold the breath. Try to maintain awareness throughout your yoga practice so that you regulate the flow of air.

One form of breath control recommended for yoga is ujjayi breathing, which means victorious breath. With this method, the breath is drawn in slowly through the nose, while the glottis is gently contracted, producing a soft hissing sound at the back of the throat. A simultaneous contraction of the abdomen should happen automatically. This breathing regulates and lengthens the air flow through the nostrils. It creates heat in the body, enhances flexibility, and soothes the nervous system.

SYNCHRONIZED MOVEMENTS
All yoga movements are performed in synchronization with the breath. Generally, you exhale as you bend forward and inhale as you come up and bend backward. It is indicated for most of the poses in this book when to inhale and exhale, but where there is no indication, then just breathe normally. Try to hold each pose for a minimum of eight breaths. However, to build strength and stamina, hold the poses for as long as is comfortable, without straining.

The breath can be used to direct *prana* flow and relieve tension when holding an asana. By concentrating on sending the breath into an area of discomfort, you can relax the muscles there.

The benefits of meditation

Yoga is freedom from mental disturbances.

The yoga sutras of Patanjali 1.2

All human beings, whether consciously or unconsciously, seek happiness. However, according to the yoga sutra, we are deluded or constantly disillusioned as we search for happiness outside of ourselves, through our jobs, our friends, or our possessions. External objects can provide only temporary satisfaction, for the mind is such that as soon as a desire is fulfilled the object obtained loses its attractiveness, and we begin to find faults.

There is a Sanskrit saying, "as the mind, so the man; bondage or liberation are in your own mind." The yoga sutras say that true lasting happiness, peace and serenity can only be experienced when in deep meditation. This is the definition of yoga, which is written in the sutras as "freedom from mental disturbances." When we are not distracted by the senses and our thoughts, we can find the source of our being, and experience joy and serenity.

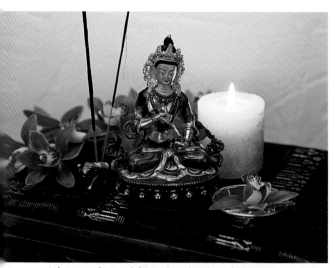

A home altar with an inspirational image, a candle, and incense can focus you on meditation.

THE INQUISITIVE MIND

The yoga scripture likens the mind to a monkey, always inquisitive, jumping from one thought to the next. *Asana* and *pranayama* practices (Steps 3 and 4 in the sutras, see p.7) begin the process of bringing the senses under control and withdrawing the mind from sense objects. This stage of drawing the mind inward is the fifth step in the yoga sutra, called *Pratyahara,* and is the beginning of raja yoga or the higher spiritual practices of meditation.

Step six is *Dharana,* which is defined as concentrating the mind in a single place. There are many meditation tools for centering the mind, such as repeating a mantra, observing the breath, or focusing on a candle or yantra (see *Meditation* p.113).

The seventh step is *Dhyana.* Initially, the mind can focus only briefly on the object of meditation, such as the breath, as it becomes easily distracted. However, with practice, the mind can fix on the object for longer periods until there is a flow in concentration—this is *Dhyana.* Physiologically the brain waves become longer, and the practitioner may experience a lightness of body and serenity.

ULTIMATE BLISS

The final stage of meditation, the eighth step, rarely attained, is *Samadhi.* Here the sense of "I", the meditator, and the object of meditation disappear. This is yoga (union), when consciousness is no longer fragmented, but is pure, devoid of subject and object. It is devoid of differentiation and the oneness is experienced as pure bliss—the eternal now.

CHAPTER 1

Warm-up
Stretches

The major asanas are physically demanding and have a powerful effect on the mind and body, so, before commencing yoga practice, it is essential that you prepare your body. Warm-up stretches help to loosen the primary joints, release residue tension in the muscles, and ease stiffness. On a subtle level, they also remove energy blocks allowing *prana* (energy) to move unhindered around the body, which gives more freedom of movement.

It is important to do the warm-up exercises gently, so that you do not strain your body. While practicing the movements, bring your awareness to the interaction of the joints, ligaments, and muscles, and observe how each movement relates to other areas of your body.

Always practice yoga on an empty stomach—allow two or three hours after your last meal. Wear comfy, stretchy clothing that will not restrict your circulation, and always use a sticky yoga mat to do the poses.

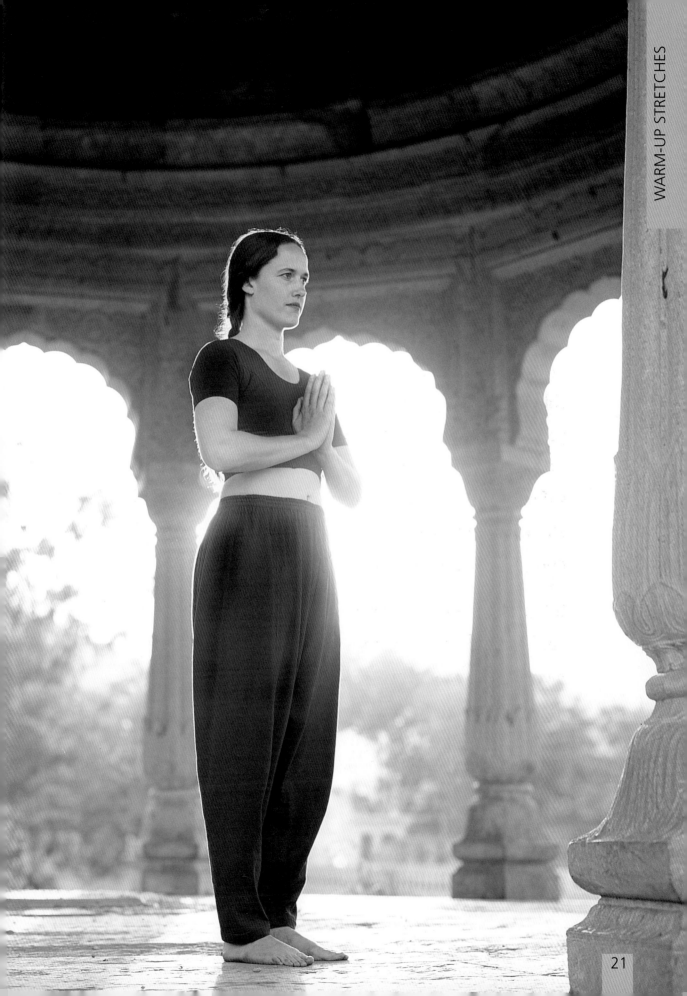

Head rolls

1 **Inhale:** sit upright in a comfortable seated position, with your arms and shoulders relaxed.
Exhale: lower your chin down toward your sternum.

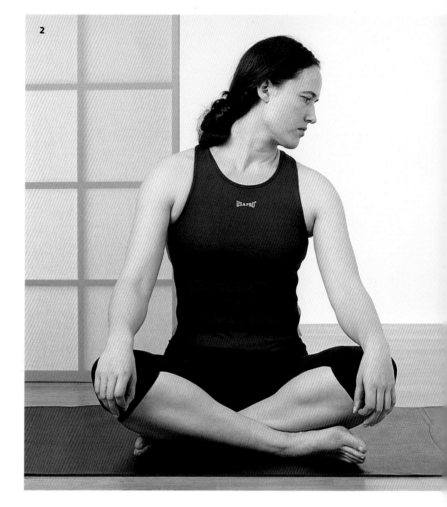

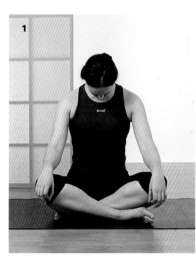

2 **Inhale:** gently roll your head up and to the side to look over your left shoulder. Make the movement as soft and fluid as possible.

3 Continue to roll your head up on the inhalation to look up toward the ceiling. Make sure that your shoulder blades are relaxed down your back.

4 **Exhale:** slowly drop your head to the opposite side to look over your right shoulder. Continue to roll your head down and back to the first position.

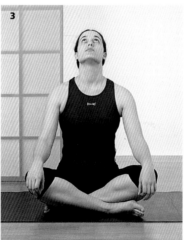

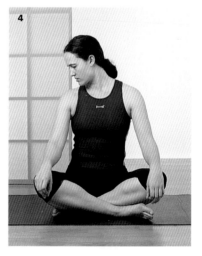

Repeat the exercise twice in one direction and twice in the opposite direction. If you find some discomfort in your neck, rest in that position briefly and breathe into the area to release the tension.

Sitting side stretch

1 Sit upright in a comfortable cross-legged position. Place your right hand on the mat about 1¹/₂ ft/45 cm from your right hip with your fingers pointing toward the end of the mat.

2 Rotate your left arm until your palm is facing the ceiling.
Inhale: lift your left arm up and over your head to the right, so that you feel the stretch along the entire left side of your body.
Exhale: keep your left 'sit' bones (in your buttocks) firmly grounded on the floor as you stay in the stretch.
Breath: hold the pose for eight or more breaths. Release the pose and repeat on the other side.

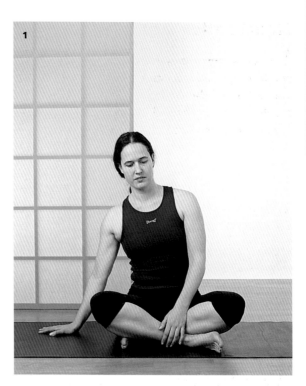

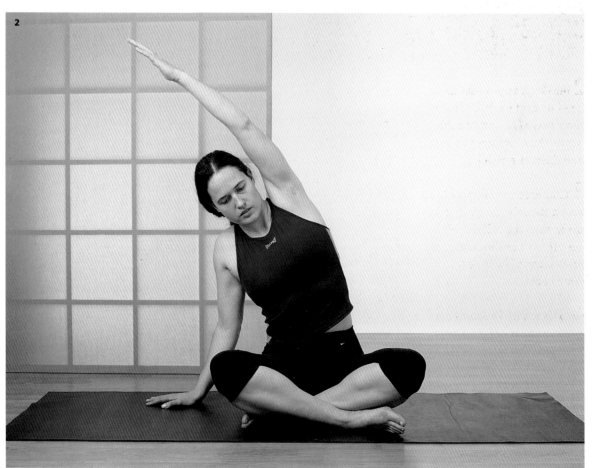

Sitting forward stretch

1 Sit upright in a comfortable cross-legged position on the mat.
Inhale: lean forward and place your hands on the mat about 1¹⁄₂ ft/45 cm in front of you.

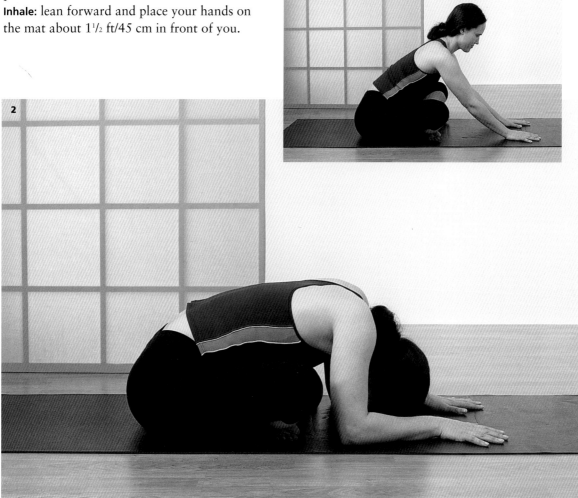

2 **Exhale:** slowly bend your elbows backward so that your arms rest on the mat, and drop your head forward until your forehead touches the mat. Gently round your spine and release any tension in your head and neck. Keep your sit bones pressing down toward the floor.
Breath: keep breathing evenly for eight breaths. Release the pose.

HELPFUL HINTS

■ If your head does not touch the floor then place a block underneath your head, or try a folded blanket.

■ While in the posture, take your awareness to your spine. Visualize your breath moving up and down the length of your spinal column so that you remove tension and increase the flexibility in your back.

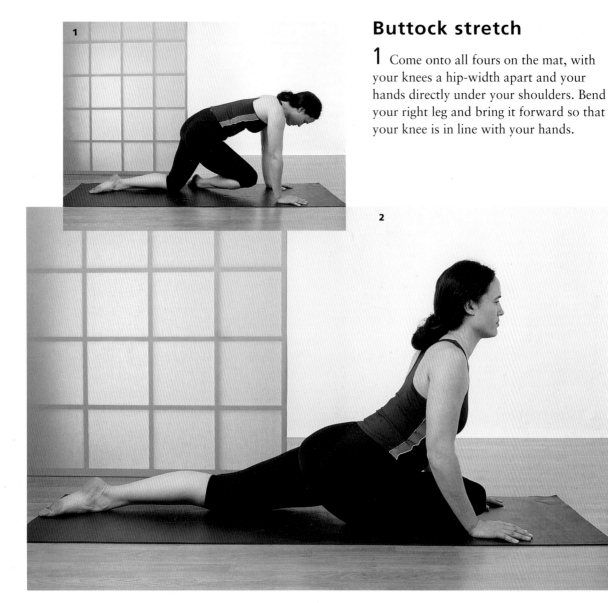

Buttock stretch

1 Come onto all fours on the mat, with your knees a hip-width apart and your hands directly under your shoulders. Bend your right leg and bring it forward so that your knee is in line with your hands.

2 **Inhale:** bend your right knee slightly to the side so that your right heel is in line with your left hip. Stretch your left leg out behind you and point your toes out and away.

3 **Exhale:** bend your elbows back and drop your forehead toward the floor. Keep your left leg stretched behind you, and drop your left hip toward your right heel.
Breath: keep breathing evenly in this pose for eight or more breaths. Release the pose and repeat on the other side.

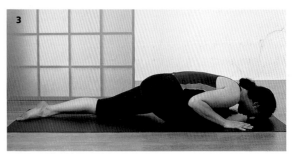

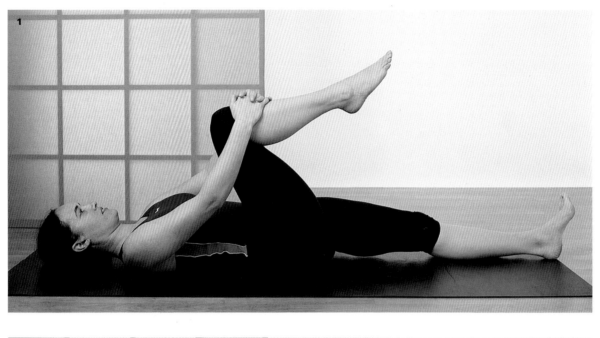

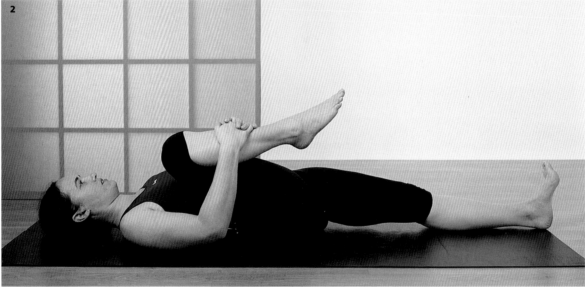

One knee to chest

1 Lie flat on your back on the mat, with your feet together. Raise your right leg and then bend your knee. Clasp both your hands firmly around your shin, just below the knee.

2 **Inhale:** take a deep breath in.
Exhale: hug your bent leg close to your chest. Keep your straight leg strong by pushing into your left heel. Try to push your tailbone (coccyx) down toward the floor. Relax your head and neck and make sure there is no tension in your jaw.
Breath: keep breathing evenly for eight or more breaths. Release the pose and repeat on the other side.

One knee to the side

1 **Inhale:** lie flat on your back with your feet together. Raise your left leg and bend your knee. Hold your leg just below the knee with your left hand.

2 **Exhale:** draw your knee close to your chest and then drop your knee out to the left side, rotating it from the hip. Keep your right leg strong by pushing into your heel and drawing your toes toward you. **Breath:** keep breathing evenly for eight or more breaths. Release the pose and repeat on the other side.

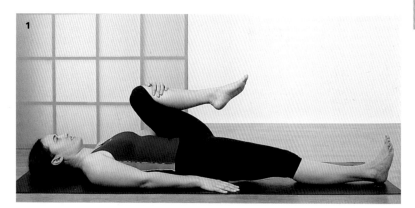

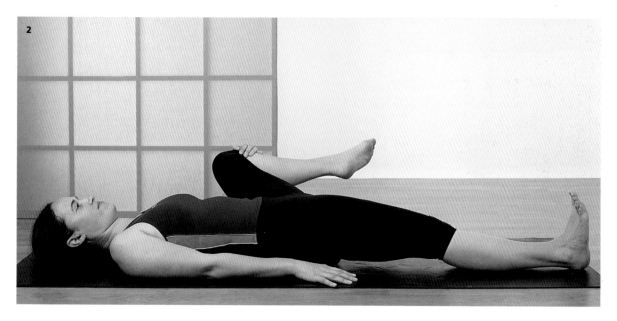

BENEFITS

■ Bringing your knees to the chest is a very useful exercise for relieving the pain of backache or sciatica as it creates traction along the spine.

■ Taking the knee to the side helps to loosen the hip joints.

■ Both exercises are excellent poses for helping digestive problems, such as releasing colic, and toning the lower intestines.

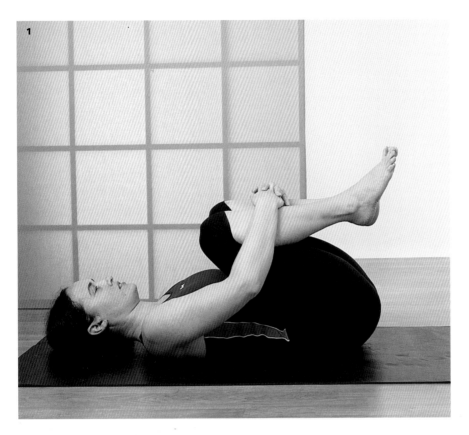

Head to knees

1 Lie flat on your back on the mat with your feet together.
Inhale: raise both legs up and bend your knees, then clasp both your hands around your shins.

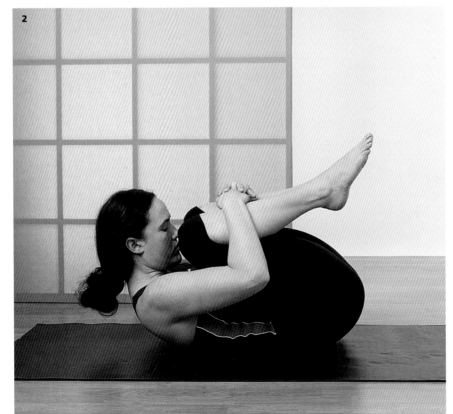

2 **Exhale:** hug your bent legs close to your chest. Try to keep your tailbone (coccyx) on the floor.
Inhale: hold the position briefly.
Exhale: lift your forehead toward your knees.
Breath: hold the pose for five breaths. Release the pose.

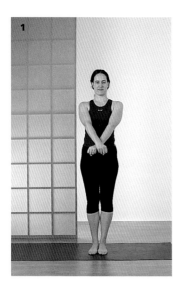

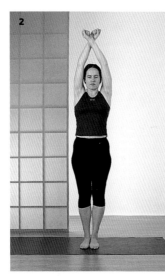

Arm circles

1 Stand upright in *tadasana* pose (see p.38) with your feet together. Make loose fists with your hands and cross your arms at your wrists.

2 Inhale: slowly rotate your arms up and over your head. Try to keep your shoulders relaxed.

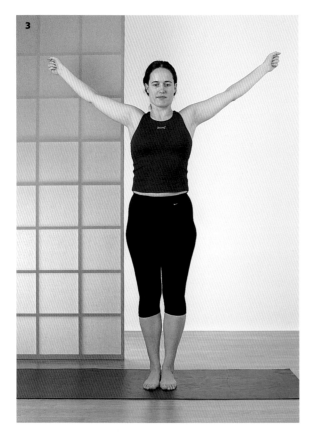

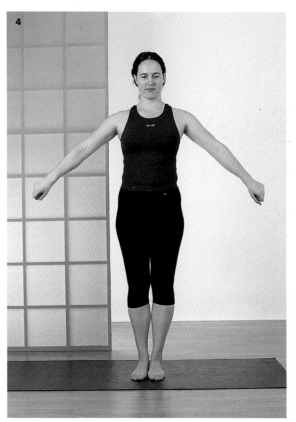

3 Exhale: continue the rotation, allowing your arms to move out naturally to the sides. Continue to rotate your arms back and out to the sides, moving all the way around until you are back to the first position.
Breath: keep breathing evenly.

4 Repeat the rotation at least twice in one direction and twice in the opposite direction. In the opposite direction, rotate your arms backward and cross your wrists above your head to come forward again.

Cat stretch

1 Move from a kneeling position on the mat to come up on all fours. Place your hands directly under your shoulders with your middle fingers pointing forward. Place your knees in line with your hips 1 ft/30 cm apart, with your toes pointing backward.

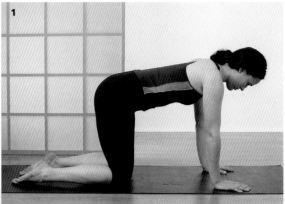

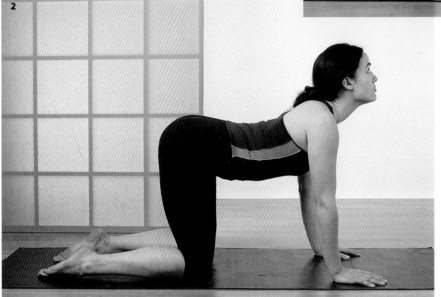

2 **Inhale:** Lift your tailbone (coccyx) and sacrum toward the ceiling, making your lower back concave, until your head lifts naturally toward the ceiling.

3 **Exhale:** tuck your tail under and arch your back toward the ceiling, allowing the action in the lower back to initiate the movement through the upper spine. Tuck your head in, pointing your chin toward your sternum. Repeat up to ten times in slow rhythmic motions in time with your breathing.

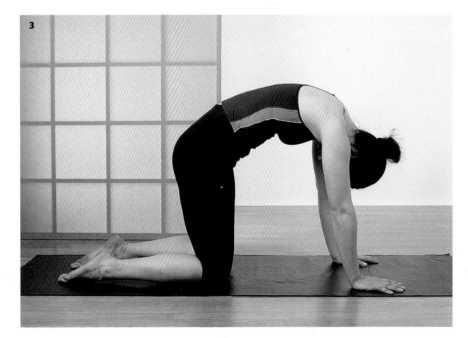

Lunge

1 Kneel with your thighs parallel. Bend your left leg and position it on the floor in front of you so that it forms a right angle. Keep your spine straight and place a hand on top of your left knee.

2 With both hands on your left knee, lunge forward by increasing the bend in your left knee. Tuck your tailbone under and drop your right thigh and groin toward the floor. Keep your head and chest lifted.

Breath: keep breathing evenly for eight or more breaths. Release the pose and repeat on the other side.

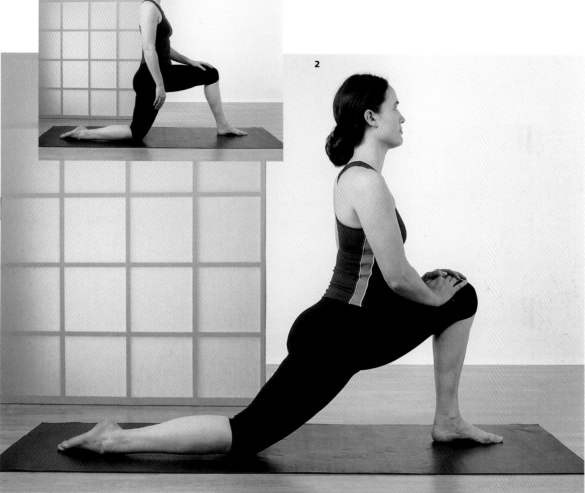

BENEFITS

■ The cat stretch increases flexibility in the spine, neck and shoulders and gently tones the female reproductive system.

■ The lunge stretches the thigh muscles and opens out the groin, allowing a fresh blood supply into these areas.

surya namaskar

Sun salutation

Surya namaskar is a dynamic series of fourteen asanas that are linked together with the breath. The flow of each asana helps to create heat in the body, which limbers up the spine and tones the joints, muscles, and internal organs. The sun salutation series regulates the solar plexus or *pingala nadi* that conducts vitality and energy through the body.

1 Stand upright in *tadasana* pose (see p.38) at the front of the mat with your feet together, and your hands together in prayer pose—*namaste*.

2 **Inhale:** stretch your arms up, interlock your hands and point upward with your index fingers so that your feel the stretch evenly along both sides of your body. Look up toward your thumbs, without tipping your head too far back.

3 Lift your chest toward the ceiling to open your heart center. Do not strain your lower back.

4 **Exhale:** bend forward from your hips, keeping your back and knees straight. Relax your head down toward your knees and put your hands on the mat next to your feet. If your hands do not quite touch the floor then bend your knees.

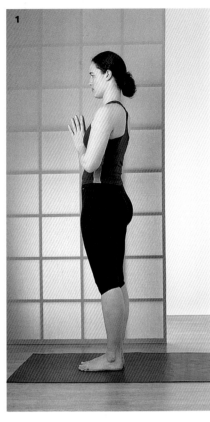

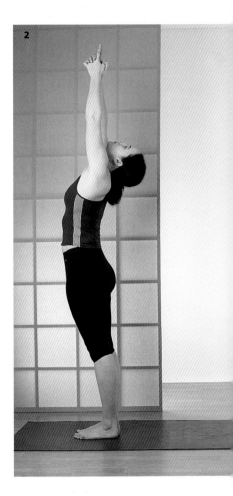

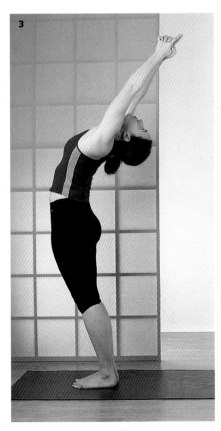

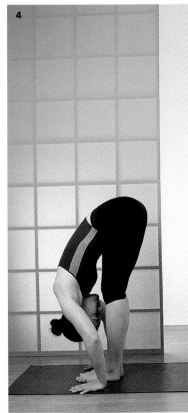

5 Inhale: stretch your left leg out behind you and drop your left knee to the floor. Move your chest forward and look up.

6 Come up onto your toes and take your right foot back in line with your left. Lower your buttocks so that your back is in one inclined plane, with your head in line with your spine.
Breath: keep holding the breath.

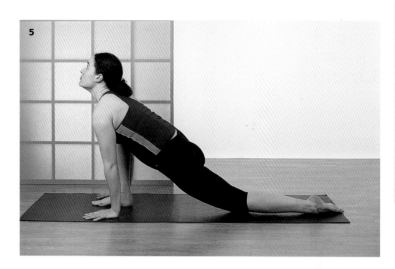

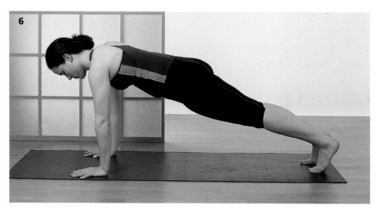

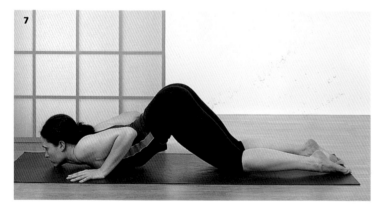

7 Exhale: bend your knees to the floor and lower your chest to the floor between your bent arms and hands, leaving your pelvis raised. Place your chin on the floor.

8 Inhale: tuck your tailbone under and slide your body weight forward. Press down into the palms of your hands and stretch out your spine, lifting up your head, neck, and chest. Look up toward the ceiling, but make sure your pelvis is still on the floor.

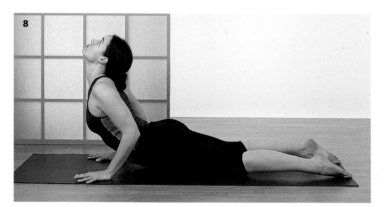

Sun salutation (continued)

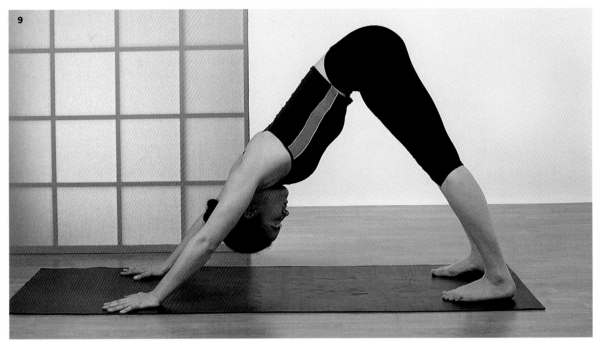

9

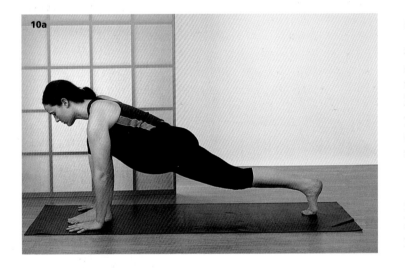

10a

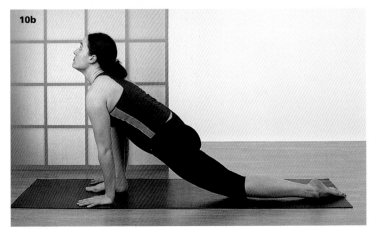

10b

9 **Exhale:** push into your hands, raise your buttocks up into the air and back so that your body forms a triangle. Relax the crown of your head toward the floor and release your neck. Keep lengthening the spine and press your heels toward the floor.

10a **Inhale:** lift your left leg forward, in line with your hands. Bend your right knee and release your pelvis down.

10b Lift your chest forward, lengthen the spine, and look up.

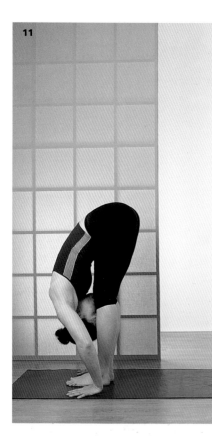

11 **Exhale:** come into forward bend by bringing your right foot forward to line up with your left foot. Lift up your thighs and straighten through the backs of your legs. Relax your head down toward your knees.

12 **Inhale:** flatten your back, reach up, and out until you are back at Step 3.

13 Release the stretch and return to Step 2.

14 **Exhale:** bring your hands back down in front of your chest. **Inhale:** repeat the cycle, taking your right leg back first to complete one full round of *surya namaskar*.

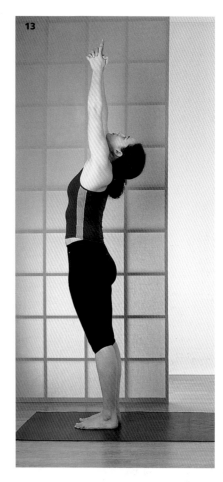

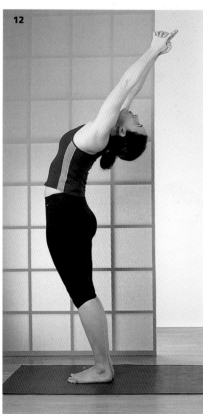

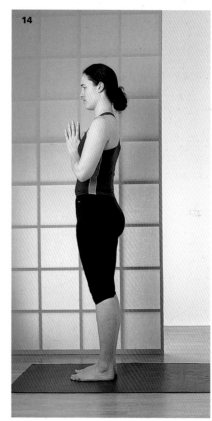

35

CHAPTER 2

Standing
Poses

Standing poses lay a firm foundation for the more advanced poses. More importantly, they teach us to stand on our own two feet, building confidence, poise, and grace. Because of the rotational and bending motion of the standing poses, the major joints of the body are lubricated, the skeletal structure is re-aligned, and body circulation improved. These poses are particularly beneficial for people suffering from arthritis and rheumatism. They are great for people with desk jobs who sit for most of the day and who really need to stretch out their bodies. For greater comfort, it is advisable always to practice the standing pose on a sticky mat or other non-slip surface.

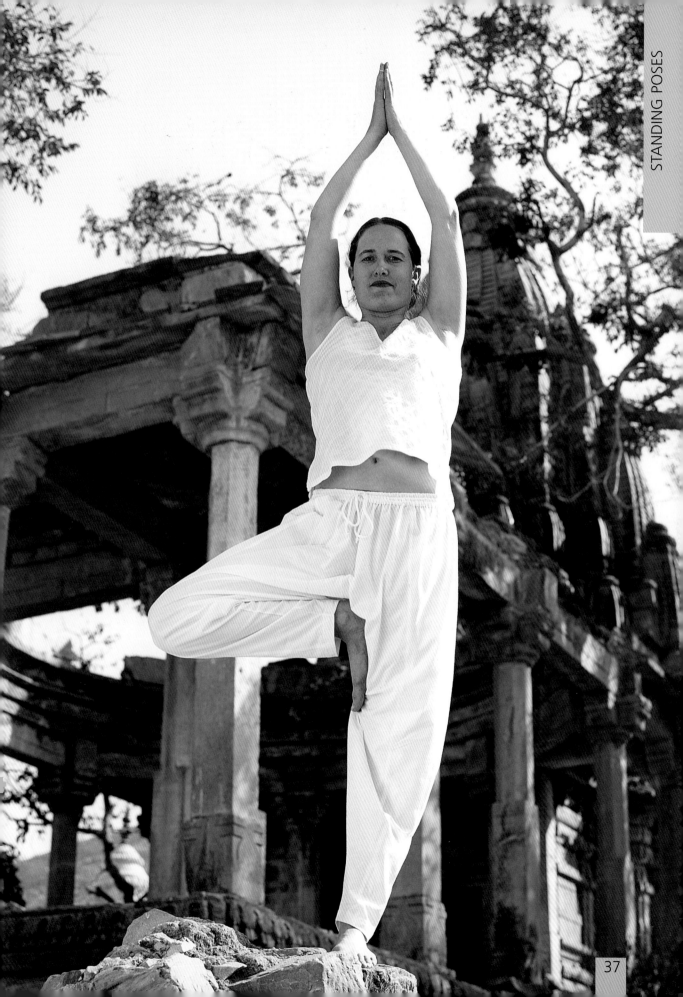

tadasana

Mountain pose

Tadasana teaches you how to achieve balance and steady the mind. Always return to *tadasana* between standing poses to center your mind.

Stand with your feet together but with your toes spread apart. Distribute your weight evenly on both feet and lift up from the inner arches. Stand straight, and lift your knees by pulling up your thigh muscles. Make sure your hips are positioned over your ankles with your tailbone tucked under slightly. Open your chest by moving your shoulders up, back, and down—relax your shoulders and keep them in line with your hips. Keep your arms hanging loosely each side of your body. Tuck your chin in slightly and extend the back of your neck. Feel the lower half of your body from your navel down rooted into the ground, and feel the upper body from your navel up lifting up toward the heavens.
Breath: keep breathing evenly for eight or more breaths.

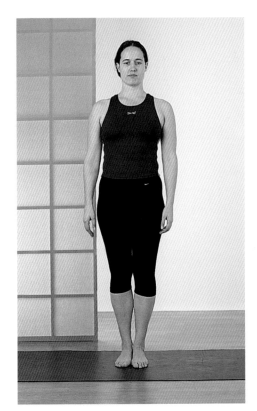

Jumping

Jumping is an optional transition between standing poses. Jumping produces lightness and agility in the body and exhilarates the mind.

1 Stand upright in *tadasana*, then bend and raise your arms up to shoulder height with your forearms parallel.

2 **Inhale:** jump your feet to the desired width apart (depending on the pose), bring your arms above your head to give height and momentum.
Exhale: land with your feet parallel and your arms stretched out to the side at shoulder height.

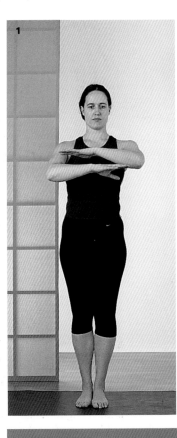

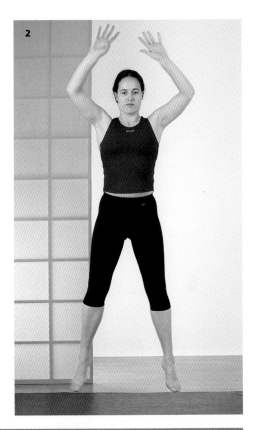

WARNING

For people who have weak backs or who suffer from knee injuries, it is advisable to step between poses.

Trikonasana

Triangle pose

1 Stand with your feet 3–4 ft/1–1.2 m apart with your arms extended at shoulder height, palms facing the floor. Relax your shoulders and pull your kneecaps up by tightening your thigh muscles.

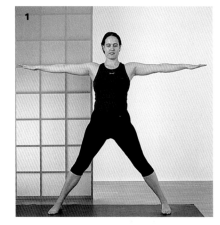

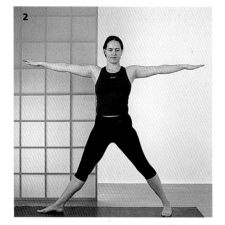

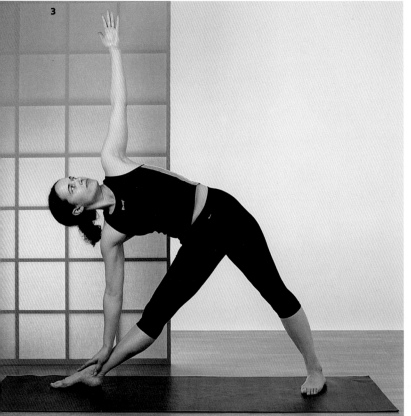

2 Turn your right leg out so that your right foot points toward the end of the mat, keeping your knee in line with your ankle. Turn your left foot in slightly toward the right, keeping your instep in line with your right heel.

3 **Inhale** and as you **exhale**: bend sideways to the right, placing your right hand on your ankle, the floor or your leg as far you can reach. Lift your left arm up to the ceiling and turn your head to look up toward your left thumb. Keep your left hip lifted, and rotate your chest up so that your body is in a straight line. **Breath**: keep breathing steadily for at least eight breaths. Release the pose and repeat on the other side.

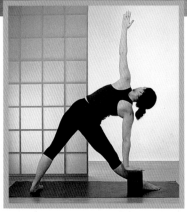

■ BEGINNER'S VERSION

Many beginners find it difficult to reach down to the side to touch the floor or their ankle without losing the integrity of the pose. So practice this pose using a block. Position the block by your ankle or calf so that you can easily place your hand on it in Step 3.

parivrtta trikonasana

Reverse triangle pose

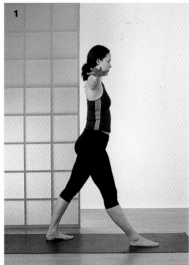

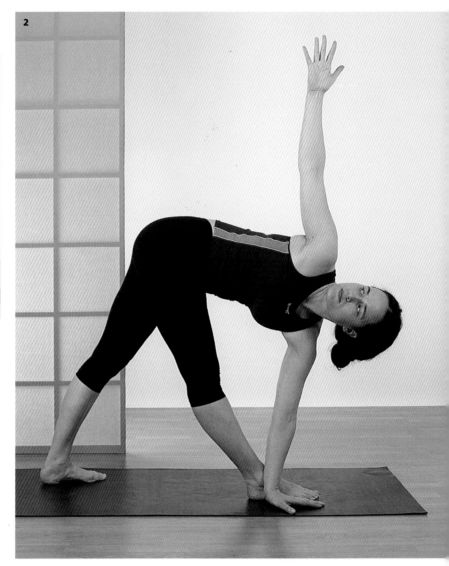

1 **Inhale:** jump so that your feet are 3–4 ft/1–1.2 m apart with your arms stretched out to the sides. Turn your feet and torso to the right so that you face the end of the mat. Engage your thigh muscles. Keep your legs strong and your feet firmly grounded.

2 **Exhale:** pivot from your hips and lean down to place your left hand on the outside of your right foot. Rotate your hips, extend your chest, and lift your right arm in the air. Look up toward your extended right arm. Use the pressure between your wrist and ankle to maintain the balance and to turn your torso more.
Breath: keep breathing evenly for eight or more breaths. Release the pose and repeat on other side.

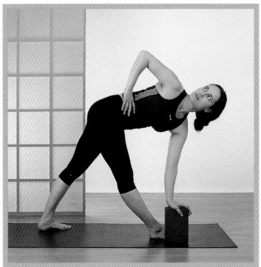

■ **BEGINNER'S VERSION**
Reaching the floor with your hand and maintaining the balance in this pose is very difficult for beginners. To help you practice this pose, place your left hand on an upright block in Step 2, and put your right hand on your hip. Concentrate on rotating and lifting your upper shoulder.

parsvakonasana

Extended side stretch

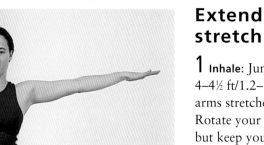

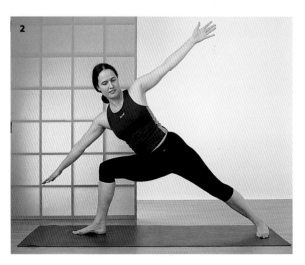

1 **Inhale:** Jump so that your feet are 4–4½ ft/1.2–1.3 m apart with your arms stretched out to the sides. Rotate your right leg and foot 90° but keep your hips facing forward. Bend your right knee until it is over the ankle, turning left foot in slightly.

2 **Exhale:** lean over to the right and place your right hand on the outside of your right foot with your fingers in line with your toes. Keep your feet grounded and maintain pressure along the outside of your left foot. Keep the thigh of your bent leg parallel with the mat edge.

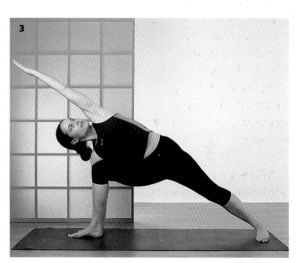

■ BEGINNER'S VERSION

If you find it difficult as a beginner to reach the floor without slumping over your bent leg, then place your hand on top of a block as you stretch in Step 3.

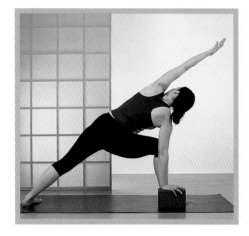

3 Rotate your left arm in its socket until the palm faces the ceiling. Then extend it out in line with your left ear so that it forms a diagonal line along the left of your body from the heel to your fingertips. Turn your head and look up to the hand.
Breath: keep breathing evenly for eight or more breaths. Release the pose and repeat on opposite side.

parivrtta parsvakonasana

Reverse extended side stretch

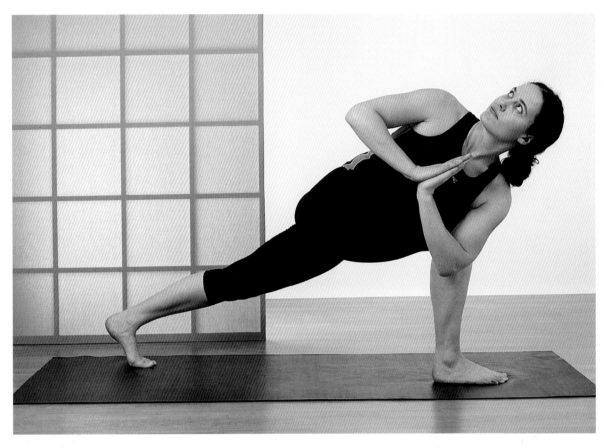

Inhale: jump so that your feet are 4–4½ ft/ 1.2–1.3 m apart with your arms stretched out to the side. Rotate your feet, legs and torso to the right side, to face the end of the mat. Bend your right leg so that it forms a right angle.

Exhale: rotate and bend the left side of your body toward your right leg. Move your left arm so that your armpit is outside your right knee. Use the pressure of your right upper arm against your right leg to rotate your torso. Bring your hands together in prayer position – *namaste* – in the center of your chest and look up to the ceiling. Come up onto the toes of your left foot, but extend into your left heel to strengthen your back leg.

Breath: keep breathing evenly for eight or more breaths. Release the pose and repeat on other side.

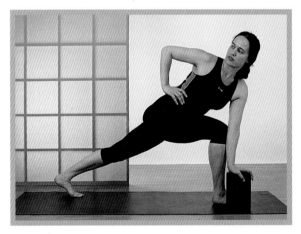

■ BEGINNER'S VERSION

To make this position easier as a beginner, place a block by the foot of your bent leg. Bend down and place your left hand on top of the block. Keep your right hand on your hip and continue rotating your top shoulder back. Make sure that your head is in line with your spine.

padottanasana

Extended leg pose

1 **Inhale:** jump so that your feet are 4–4½ft/1.2–1.3 m apart and place your hands on your hips. Keep your feet parallel and your legs strong. Tuck your tailbone under slightly and stretch out your chest.

2 **Exhale:** bend forward keeping your back flat and place your hands on the floor directly under your shoulders on the edge of the mat. Keep your hips in line with your heels and extend your torso from the sit bones (near your hip bones) to the top of your head. **Breath:** keep breathing evenly for eight or more breaths.

3 **Inhale,** then as you **exhale:** put your hands so that they are in line with your feet with your fingers facing forward. Bend your elbows back and take the crown of your head toward the floor between your hands. Relax your upper body and keep your legs strong. **Breath:** maintain the pose for at least eight breaths.

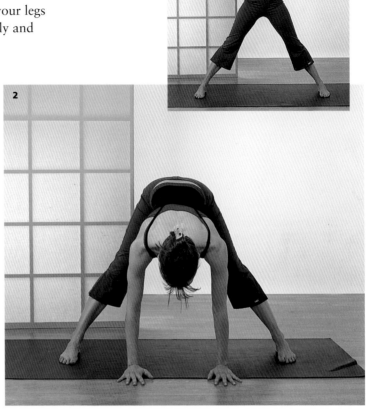

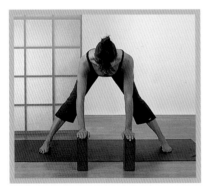

■ **BEGINNER'S VERSION**
It is difficult for beginners to bend forward and maintain a straight back. So in Step 2, place your hands on two blocks and focus on stretching out your spine.

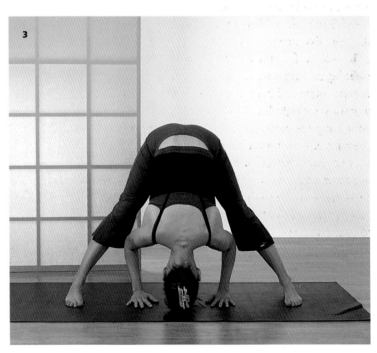

ardha chandrasana

Half moon pose

1 **Inhale:** jump so that your feet are 3–4 ft/ 1–1.2 m apart. Turn your right leg and foot out toward the end of the mat and turn your back left foot in slightly. **Exhale:** bend sideways into *trikonasana* (see p.39). Remain in the pose for a few breaths.

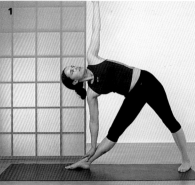

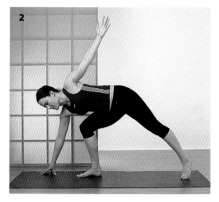

2 **Inhale**, then **exhale:** bend your right leg and place the fingertips of your right hand on the floor about 1½ft/45 cm in front of your right foot. Keep your left arm in the air, and draw your left foot in.

3 At the same time, straighten your right leg and lift your left leg up until it is parallel with the floor. Take your left arm up so that both arms form a straight line. Keep rotating your chest and lifting your left hip so that your body is on one plane. Stretch into your left heel. Turn your head to look up at your left thumb. Maintain your weight on your standing leg, not your arm. **Breath:** keep breathing steadily for eight or more breaths. Release the pose and repeat on the other side.

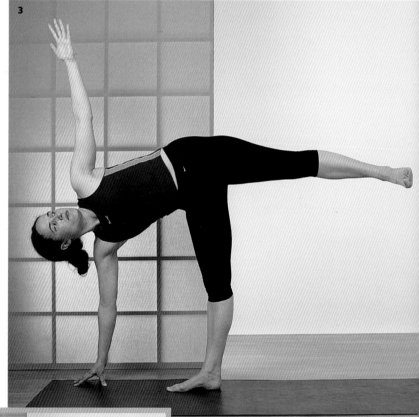

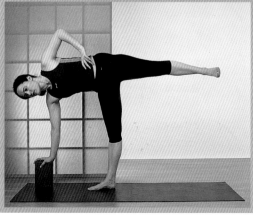

■ BEGINNER'S VERSION

To make it easier as a beginner, in Steps 2 and 3, place a block under your right hand, put your left hand on your hip and focus on rotating your left shoulder back. To help you balance, keep your eyes down on the floor or practice the pose with your back against a wall.

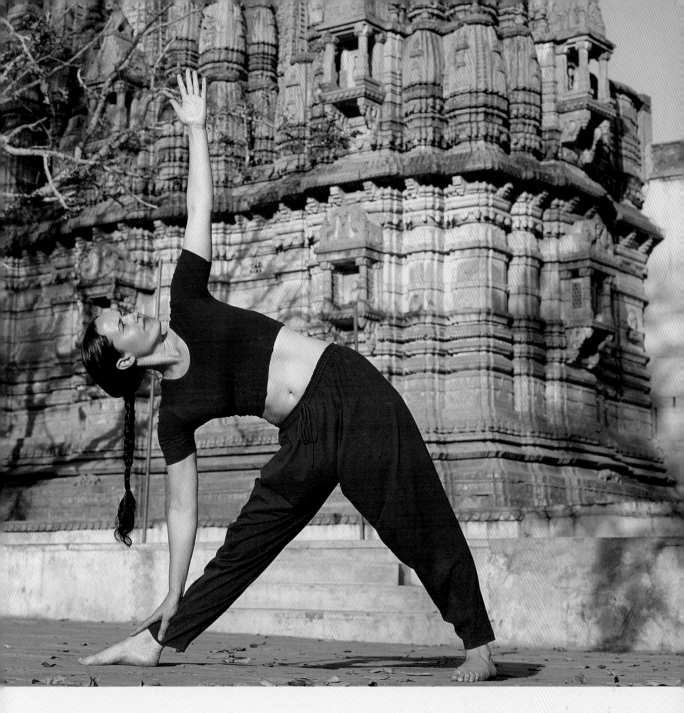

BENEFITS

- *Trikonasana* improves flexibility in the spine, and alleviates back and neck pain. It massages and tones the pelvis and abdomen, relieving indigestion and flatulence.

- *Ardha chandrasana* improves concentration and balance, bringing agility and lightness to the body. It also relieves backache and sciatica, and the pose helps to correct a prolapsed uterus.

parsvottanasana

Sideways extended pose

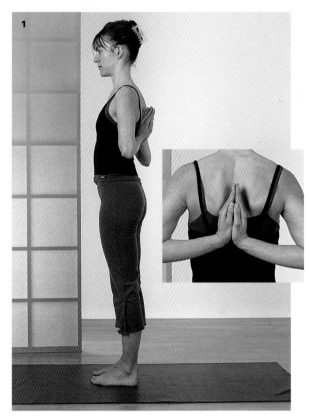

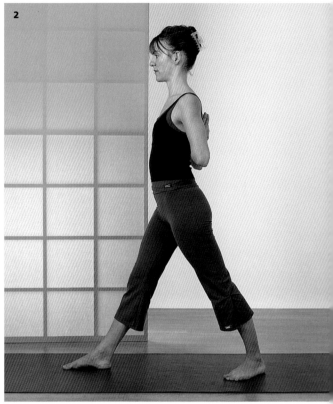

Parsvottanasana helps to work the body in several ways. Done on its own (see Step 1) it prepares the body for back bending. The forward bend (Steps 2 and 3) stretches the inner hamstrings allowing for greater mobility, whereas the separate balance pose develops concentration and poise.

1 Stand upright in *tadasana* pose (see p.38) and bring your palms together behind your back with your fingers pointing downwards. Rotate your palms by pointing your fingertips toward your back and then up, joining your palms together between your shoulder blades. Move your shoulder blades back so that you open the front of your chest. Keep your elbows back in line with your palms.

2 Inhale: step your left foot back 3–3½ ft/1–1.1 m. Keep your hips facing forward, and draw energy up from your feet by lifting your arches, and strengthening your thighs.

■ BEGINNER'S VERSION

Bringing your palms together behind you and bending forward with a flat back is difficult for beginners. So practice this pose from Step 2 and 3 balancing on two blocks, and focus on lengthening your spine and gently stretching your hamstrings.

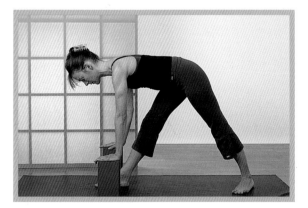

46

3 **Exhale:** bend forward with a straight back over your right leg, taking your chin toward your knee. Keep your chest in line with the middle of your right leg, and lift your elbows back, and push your palms together.
Breath: keep breathing evenly for eight or more breaths.
Inhale: come up, step your feet together, exhale and repeat on the other side.

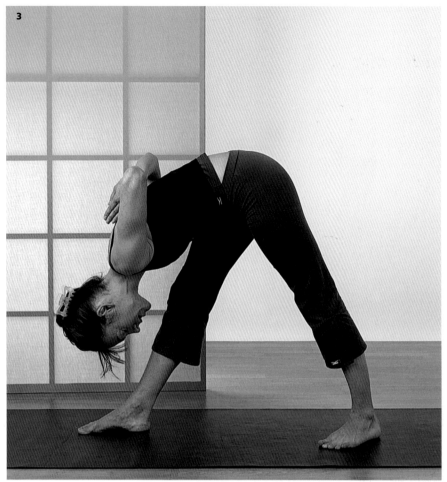

Sideways extended and balance pose

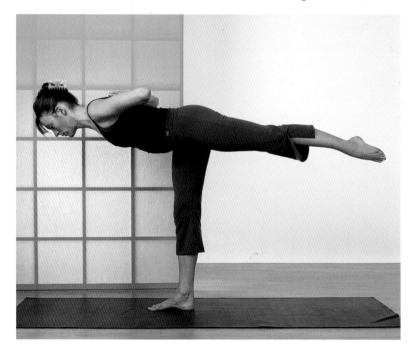

This variation of *parsvottanasana* also helps to improve balance, purify the nervous system and concentrate the mind.

From Step 2 of *Parsvottanasana* bend forward over your right leg, and, at the same time, lift your left leg up and back to form a straight line from the crown of your head to your toes. Keep your hips on one plane and your head in line with your spine.
Breath: keep breathing evenly for eight or more breaths. Release the pose and repeat on the other side.

viRabhadRasana

Warrior

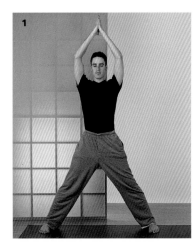

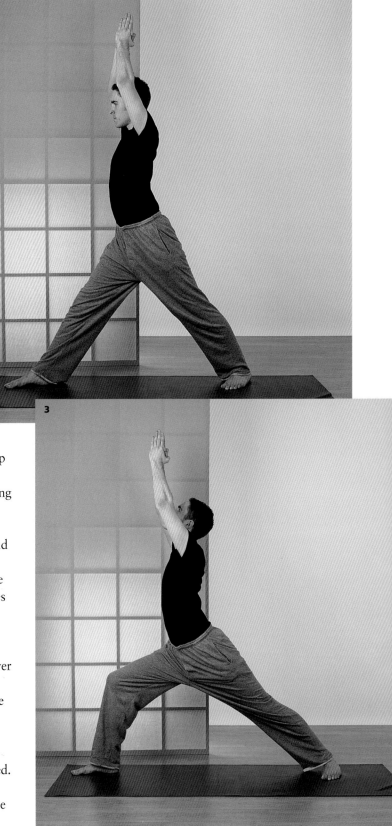

1 **Inhale:** from standing, jump so that your feet are 4–4½ ft/ 1.2–1.3 m apart and parallel. Raise your arms to shoulder height, rotate them in the sockets until your palms are facing the ceiling, and then lift them over the head until your hands are touching in prayer position. Keep your elbows straight and open your chest, taking your shoulder blades down, flattening them into your back.

2 Turn your right foot out to the right and keep your left foot turned in to face the front. Turn your body and hips to face the right. Keep your arms lifted and both sides of your body level. Both hips should be facing forward and on the same plane.

3 **Exhale:** bend your right knee until it is over your ankle. Keep your thigh parallel to the mat edge. Keep pressing on the outside edge of your left foot. Lift up your body, expanding your chest, and look up to your thumbs. Visualize the energy going to your fingertips. Keep your throat and face relaxed.
Breath: keep breathing evenly for eight or more breaths. Release the pose, turn to the center and repeat on the other side.

Warrior I

1 **Inhale:** from standing, jump so that your feet are 4–4½ ft/1.2–1.3 m apart. Stretch your arms sideways at shoulder height with the palms of your hands facing down toward the floor. Turn your right leg to face the end of the mat and your left foot in slightly to face the front. Keep your hips and torso facing forward, with your weight evenly distributed on both feet.

2 **Exhale:** bend your right leg to form a right angle, keeping your thigh parallel to the mat edge. Hold your body upright; do not allow it to lean toward your bent leg. Extend your arms from the center of your chest out to your fingertips, and relax your shoulders. Turn your head to the side to look to your right hand, pulling back with your left arm.
Breath: keep breathing evenly for about eight breaths.
Inhale: come back into the upright position, turn your feet toward the center, **exhale**, and repeat on the other side.

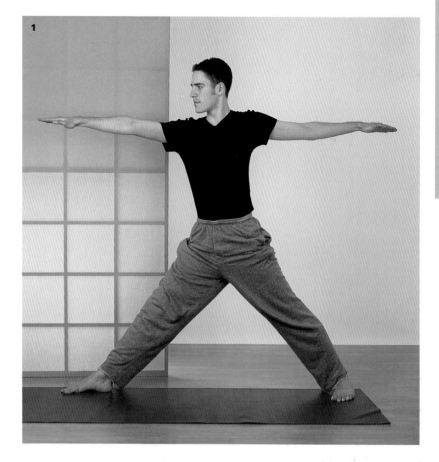

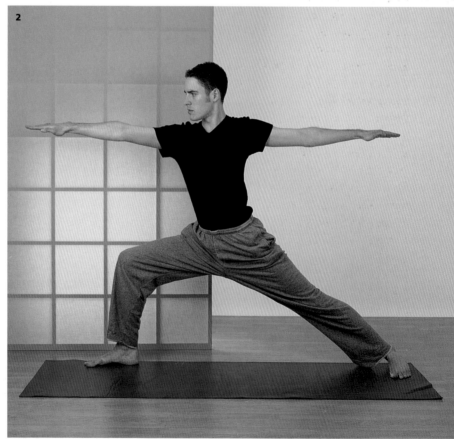

vrksasana

Tree pose

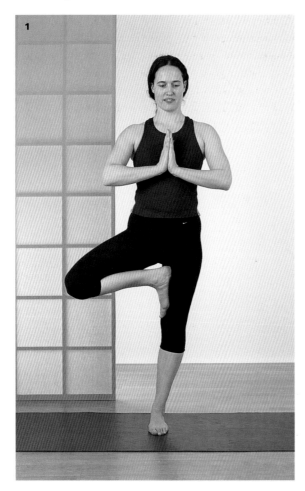

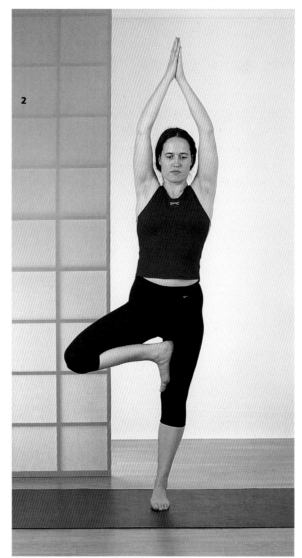

1 Stand upright in *tadasana* pose (see p.38), spread your feet and toes, and begin to take your body weight into your left leg. Raise your right leg and place the sole of your foot on the inside of your left thigh, pressing the muscles of the right leg against the sole of your foot. Bring your palms together in front of your chest.
Breath: stay in this position for eight breaths.

2 **Inhale:** raise your arms up over your head either by taking your held hands straight up or by taking your arms to the side, turning your palms up and stretching your arms over your head. Keep your shoulders blades back.
Breath: maintain the pose for eight or more breaths, and then slowly and smoothly release the pose and repeat on the other side.

HELPFUL HINTS

■ To help when you are balancing, concentrate on a spot either on the wall or about 4 ft/1.2 m in front on the floor. You can also practice the pose with your back against the wall. Keep breathing smoothly and steadily.

■ If it is difficult to raise your leg up to your inner thigh, then place it either on your stationary foot or on the inside of your stationary knee.

ūtkatasana

Powerful pose

1 **Inhale:** stand upright in *tadasana* pose (see p.38) facing to the side, and bring your feet, ankles and knees together.
Exhale: bend your legs, as if you were going to sit down on a chair. Push your hands down with your palms facing the ceiling, as if you were lifting energy up from the ground.

2 **Inhale:** bring your arms out to the sides and up, joining your palms together in front of your head.
Exhale: lift your upper body back, stretch up and look toward your thumbs. Keep your heels and feet pushing into the floor.
Breath: keep breathing evenly for eight or more breaths, then release pose.

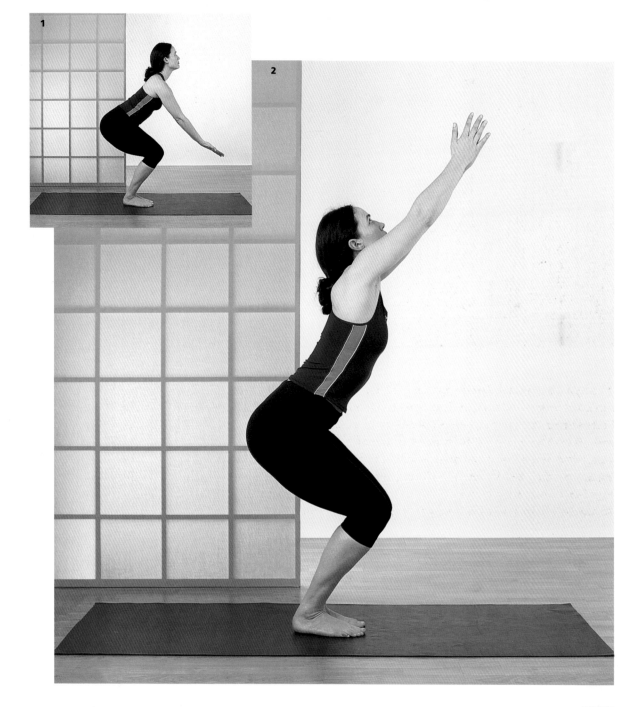

garudasana

Eagle pose

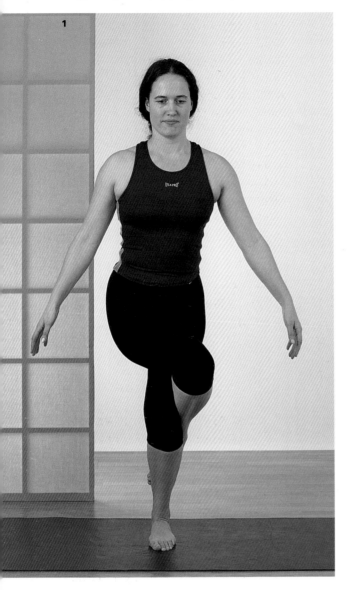

1 Stand upright in *tadasana* pose (see p.38). Slightly bend both legs and wrap your right leg around your left leg with your right thigh over your left. Take your right foot back and wrap it around your left calf. Keep your torso upright and balance with your arms out at your side. Focus on a point on the floor to maintain your balance.

2 Raise your arms and bend your elbows, keeping your forearms up and your palms facing each other. Cross your right elbow over your left. Intertwine your arms and bring your fingertips or palm of your left hand into your right. Stay balanced, looking at your point on the floor or wall. Keep your left leg slightly bent and extend your body up, with the sides of your body parallel.
Breath: keep breathing evenly for eight or more breaths. Release your arms and legs, stand straight, and repeat on the other side.

uttanasana

Forward bend

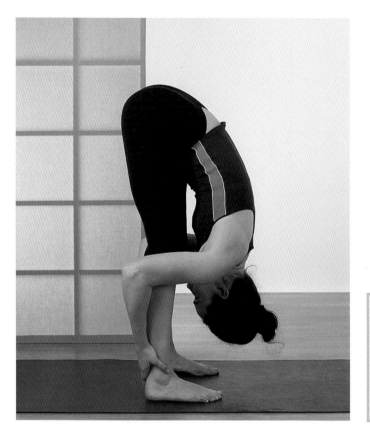

Stand upright with your feet a hip-width apart.

Inhale: raise your arms over your head.

Exhale: bend forward as far as possible without bending your knees. Clasp your hands behind your ankles and draw your face close to your knees. Keep your hips in line with your feet. Lift up the inner arches of your feet, keep your legs strong and completely relax your upper body.

Breath: remain in this pose for at least eight breaths, then release pose.

HELPFUL HINTS

■ If you suffer from lower back pain, then practice this pose with your toes turned in slightly.

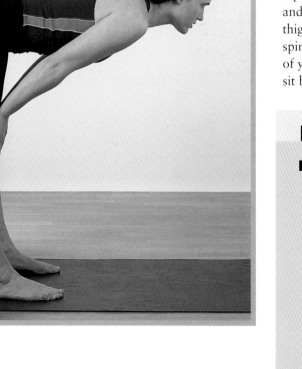

■ **BEGINNER'S VERSION**

As a beginner, you need to learn to bend forward with a straight back. Stand with your feet a hip-width apart. Bend forward and place your hands on your thighs. Focus on lengthening your spine by lifting through the backs of your legs and stretching your sit bones away from your head.

BENEFITS

■ When you do the forward bend, your heart is rested and your head receives a fresh supply of oxygen-rich blood.

CHAPTER 3
Sitting
Poses

Sitting poses are cooling, and help to calm the mind and emotions in preparation for deep meditation. They bring us in closer contact to the earth, from which we can draw strength and feel centered. The forward bends provide traction, which creates space between the vertebrae of the spine. This supplies fresh oxygen and blood to the discs and tones the back. Always ease gently into the forward bend pose so that you do not strain your back.

The poses are suitable to practice during menstruation and help regulate the flow of blood. Relaxation is the key to accomplishing the poses. If your back or hips are tight, then raise your hips up by sitting on a block or a folded blanket.

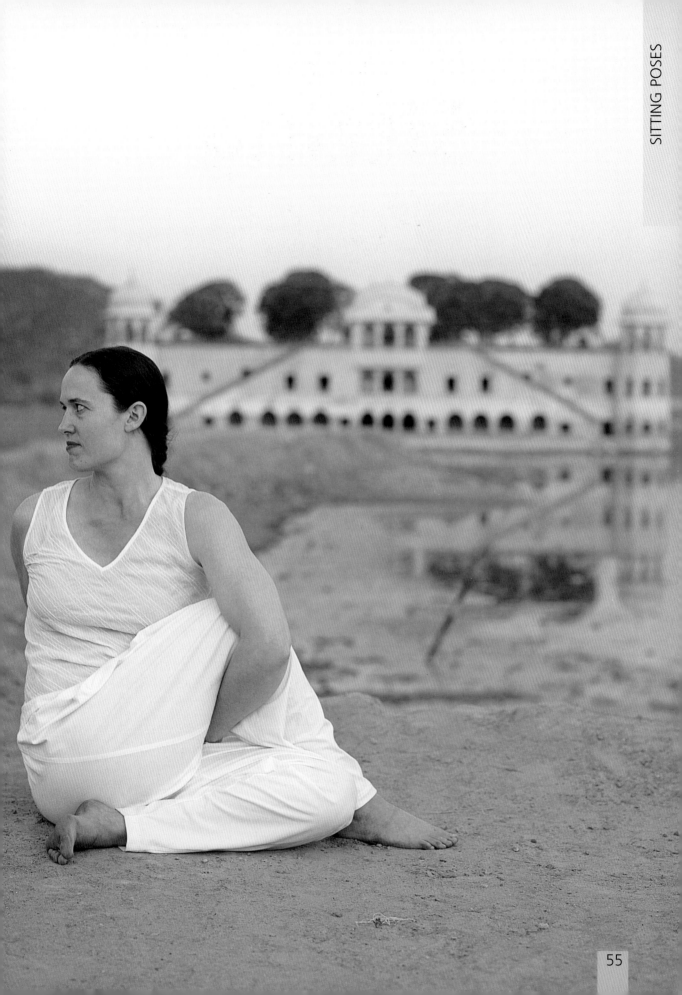

dandasana

Staff pose

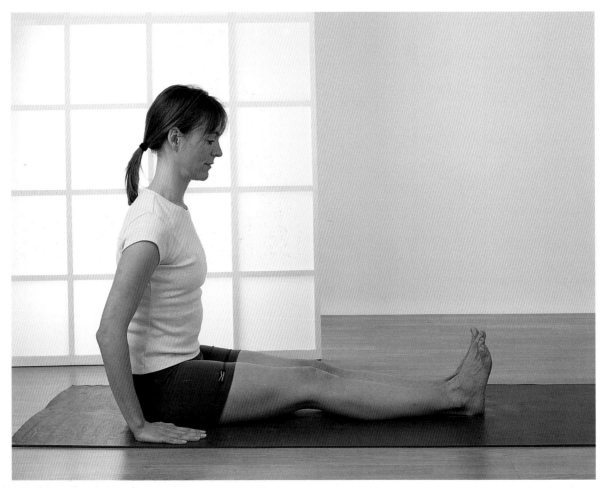

Sitting upright with your legs outstretched is called *dandasana* or staff pose. It is the neutral sitting pose to come back to for all forward bends as *tadasana* (see p.38) is for the standing poses.

1 Sit upright with an erect spine with your legs stretched out. Keep your ankles, knees, and thighs together. Push through the backs of your legs into your heels and pull up your toes. Press your thighs into the floor. Place your palms on the floor beside your hips with your fingers forward. Lift your torso up from the sit bones (near your hip bones) and draw your abdomen in and up toward your diaphragm. Open out your chest, lift up your sternum, and move your shoulders back and down. Tuck your chin in and keep your head, shoulders and hips in a line.

Breath: breathe for eight breaths, then release pose.

BENEFITS

■ Practicing this asana regularly improves your sitting posture.

■ *Dandasana* also promotes emotional stability and can relieve anxiety.

paschimottanasana

Seated forward bend

1 Sit upright in *dandasana* pose (see p.56).
Inhale: stretch your arms up over your head with your palms facing each other. Stretch up from your sit bones.
Exhale: bend forward with a flat back over your straight legs and clasp your feet with your hands or go as far down your legs as possible.
Breath: rest in this pose for a few breaths.

2 **Exhale:** take your elbows out to the sides and bring your head toward your knees. Relax the back of your neck and shoulders, and release your elbows down to the floor. Extend the sit bones away and keep the side of your body parallel. Keep your legs straight, pressing your thighs into the floor.
Breath: keep breathing evenly for eight or more breaths.
Inhale: come up, **exhale** and release the pose.

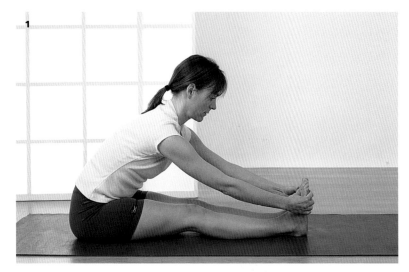

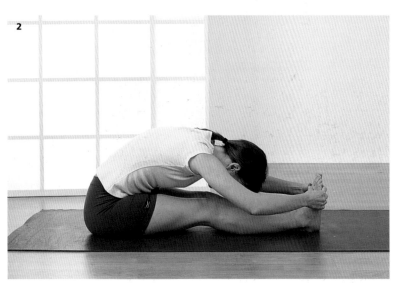

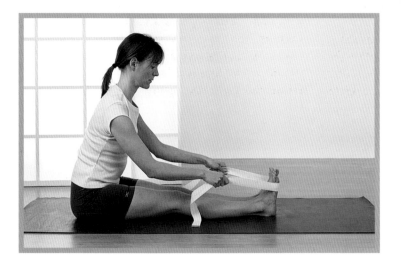

■ BEGINNER'S VERSION
Building up flexibility in the back and hamstrings requires patience and effort. If you do not find it easy as a beginner to bend forward with a flat back and touch your feet, then practice using a belt. Place a belt around your feet in Step 1, and then bend forward pulling on the belt. Only come as far forward as is comfortable. Focus on keeping your spine straight and elongating your hamstrings. Be careful not to strain in this pose.

ardha baddha padma paschimottanasana

Half-bound lotus forward bend

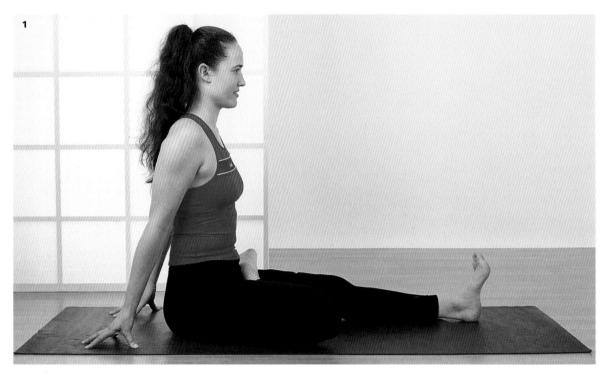

1 Sit upright in *dandasana* pose (see p.56). Bend your right leg and place your foot on top of your left thigh, close to your groin. Bring your right knee forward toward your left knee. Put your arms behind you by your hips on the mat, and balancing on your fingertips, stretch up from your sit bones (near your hip bones).

2 Take your right arm around your back so that you can take hold of your right big toe or foot (see inset). Lean forward and grasp the side of your left foot with your left hand. Gradually rotate your torso toward the center.

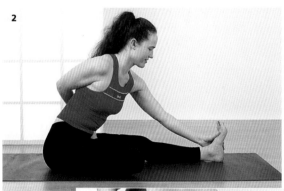

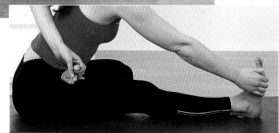

3

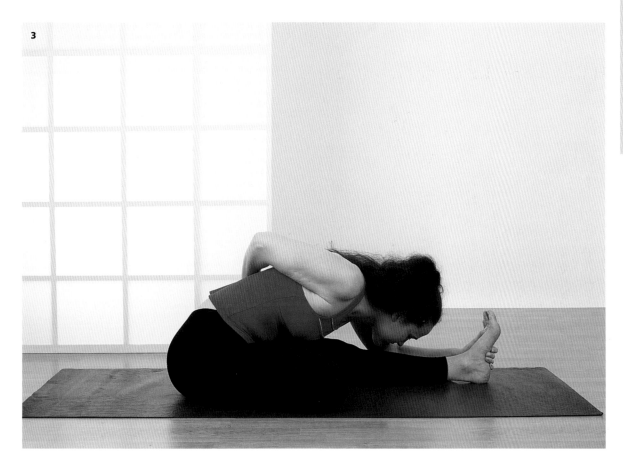

3 Exhale: bend your left elbow out to the side and lean forward over your straight leg as far as possible, taking your head or chin toward your knee. Keep your left knee straight and your left thigh pressing into the floor. Relax both your back and neck.
Breath: keep breathing evenly for eight or more breaths.
Inhale: come up, then **exhale** and repeat on the other side.

BENEFITS

■ All the forward bends tone the abdominal muscles.

■ The heel of your bent leg massages your abdomen in this pose.

■ It helps to alleviate gas, as well as toning the spine and legs muscles.

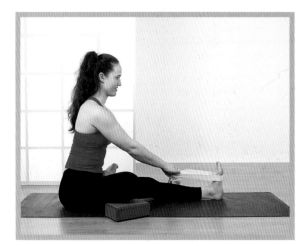

■ BEGINNER'S VERSION
Placing your leg in the half lotus pose with your knee on the floor is a difficult position for beginners. If your knee lifts off the floor, place a block or blanket under it for support. Place a belt around your left foot in the Step 2 position to help you bend forward without hunching your upper back.

triang mukhaikapada paschimottanasana

Three-pointed forward bend

1 From kneeling on the mat, start to stand on both knees. Put your left leg out in front of you and then slowly move back to sit on the inside of your right calf. Use the thumb of your right hand to move the fleshy part of your calf muscle out to the side to create more space to sit back. Keep the center of your right foot on the floor.

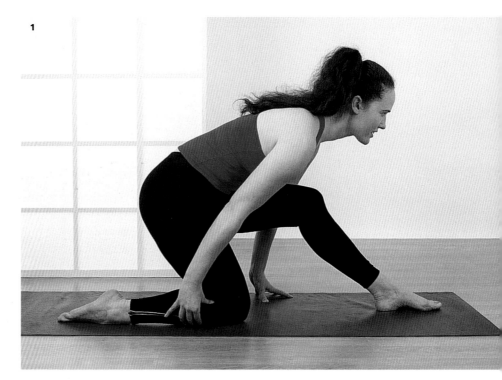

2 Straighten your left leg completely and bring both your knees together. Flex your left foot and press your left thigh into the floor. Sit upright, with your weight evenly distributed on both sit bones, and keep your hips parallel.

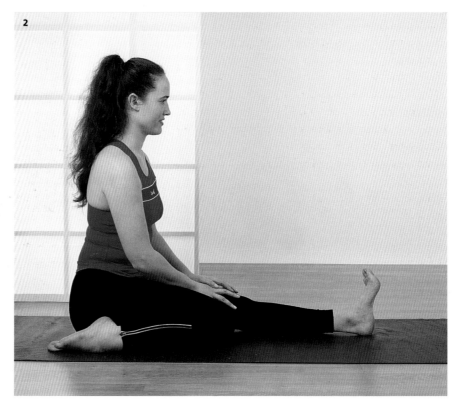

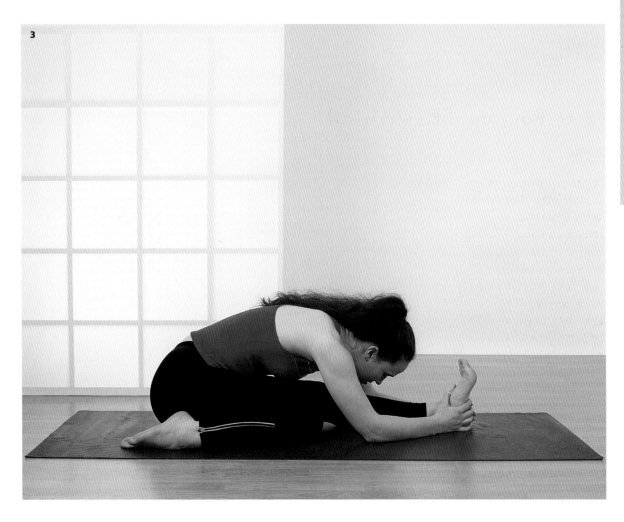

3 **Inhale:** raise your hands over your head with your palms facing each other, lifting up from your sit bones.
Exhale: bend forward over your straight leg, taking your navel toward your thigh and your head toward your knee. Hold your left foot with both your hands. Relax your neck and back, and allow your elbows to drop to the floor.
Breath: keep breathing evenly for eight or more breaths.
Inhale: come up, then **exhale** and repeat on the other side.

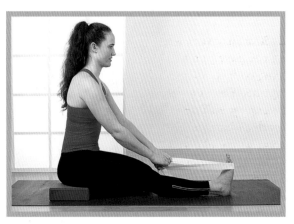

BENEFITS

- Again, this pose tones and revitalizes the abdominal organs.
- It helps to relieve compression in the spine and reduces sciatic pain.
- It makes the spine more flexible.

■ BEGINNER'S VERSION
To prevent your torso tilting toward your straight leg when you are doing this pose as a beginner, place a block or folded blanket, depending on the tilt, under the buttock of your straight leg to equalize your hips. Use a belt around your extended foot in the Step 2 position so that you can pull forward without hunching your upper back.

janu sirasana

Head to knee pose

1 Sit upright in *dandasana* pose (see p.56) with your legs straight out. Bend your right leg and place your right foot on the inside of your left thigh, with your heel close to your groin. Drop your right knee out to the side and as back as far as possible. Turn your body so that it faces the center of your extended left leg, placing both hands on your left knee.

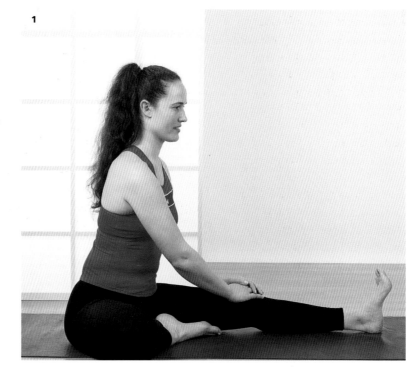

1

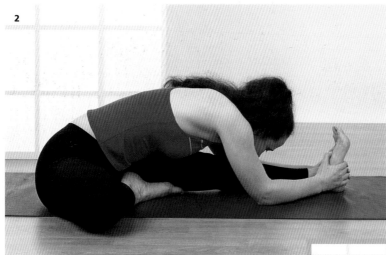

2

2 Raise your hands over your head and bend over your straight left leg to clasp your foot. Let your elbows drop out to the sides and extend your body along your leg, placing your forehead on your shin. Relax your neck and shoulders. **Breath:** keep breathing evenly for eight or more breaths. Release the pose and repeat on the other side.

■ BEGINNER'S VERSION

If your hips and back are stiff, then your knee will not touch the floor and bending forward will be difficult. In Step 1, place a block under your right knee to raise it and avoid overextension in the muscles surrounding the knee joint. To help with your forward stretch, loop a belt around the ball of your left foot and use it to pull you closer to your extended leg.

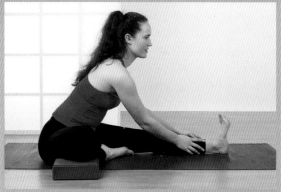

maricyasana

1 Sit upright in *dandasana* pose (see p.56). Bend your right leg, with your knee pointing upward, and place your right foot close to your right buttock by your left thigh. Keep your left leg strong, with your left thigh pressing into the mat, while your foot points upward.

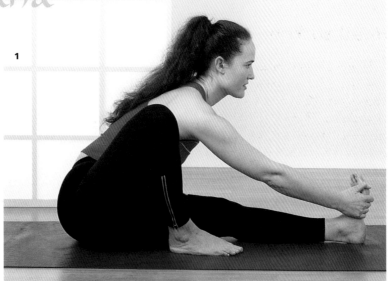

2 Bend forward over your left leg and wrap your right arm around your right bent leg toward the back with your left palm facing up. Take your left arm around your back and clasp your left hand or wrist with your right hand. Keep your head down and your body facing your left leg. Bend as far forward as possible, keeping both sides of your chest parallel and take your forehead or chin toward your left shin.
Breath: keep breathing evenly for eight or more breaths. Release the pose and repeat on the opposite side.

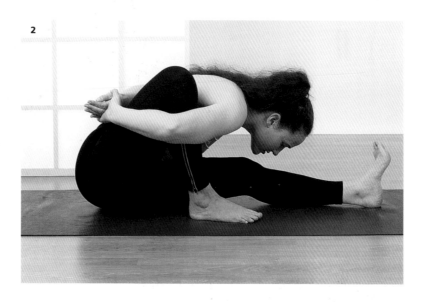

■ **BEGINNER'S VERSION**
If you find it difficult to clasp your hands behind your back, use a belt. Lay the belt loosely behind your back in Step 2 until you can grasp each end of it with your hands. Move your hands along the belt, gradually working them as close as possible together. Every time you practice the pose, try to bring your hands closer together.

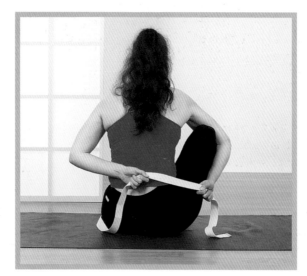

krauncasana

Heron pose

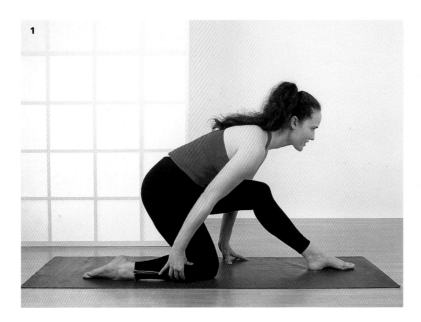

1 Sit upright in *dandasana* pose (see p.56). Bend your right leg back, using your right thumb to ease your calf muscle out to the side as in the first step of *triang mukhaikapada* (see p.60). Keep your left leg straight out in front as in *triang mukhaikapada paschimottanasana* (see p.60).

2 Sit upright with your right leg tucked to the side and keep your weight evenly balanced on your buttocks. Lean back slightly, then bend and lift your left leg, clasping both hands around the sole of your left foot.

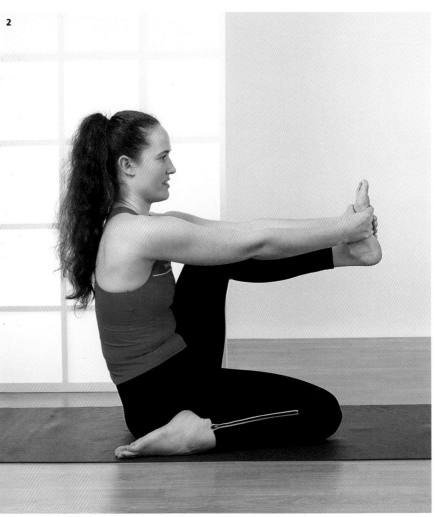

3 **Inhale:** lift up and straighten your left leg, extending throught the back of your leg into the heel, opening the back of your left knee. Straighten your arms, and extend your body upward. Keep your sternum facing the center of your raised leg.

4 **Exhale:** bend your elbows out to the side and draw your body toward your left leg. Extend your body along your raised leg and bend your head toward your left shin.

Breath: keep breathing evenly for eight or more breaths. Release, and repeat on the other side.

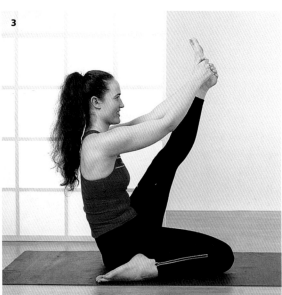

3

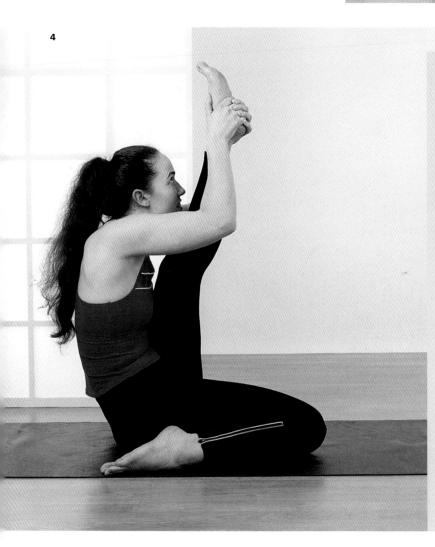

4

BENEFITS

- *Krauncasana* helps to extend the hamstring muscles and strengthens the spinal column.

- The movements also help to massage the digestive tract.

- On a subtle level this pose purifies the area from which the 72,000 *nadis* (energy channels) emanate at the base of the spine, toning the whole nervous system.

65

gomukhasana

Cow face pose

1 Sit upright in *dandasana* pose (see p.56). Bend both legs and place your feet flat on the floor about 1½ ft/45 cm from your buttocks. Pass your left leg under your right leg so that your knee is directly in front of your body with your left heel in line with your right thigh.

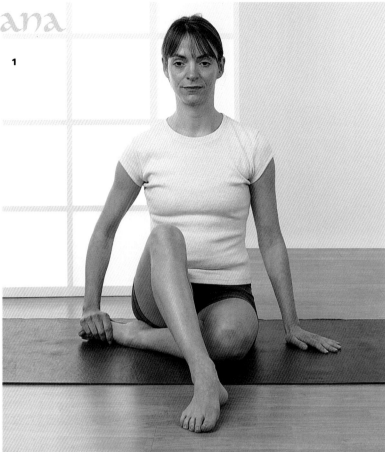

2 Cross your right leg over your left until your left knee is directly over your right knee and your right foot is by your left thigh. Stay sitting upright, between your feet, with your weight evenly distributed on your buttocks. Place your hands on top of your right knee and take a few moments to relax into the pose.

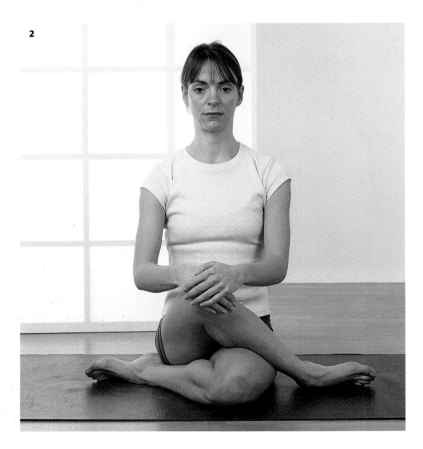

baddha konasana

Cobbler pose

1 Sit upright in *dandasana* pose (see p.56). Bend your knees and bring the soles of your feet together, close to your groin, then gently drop your knees out to the sides.

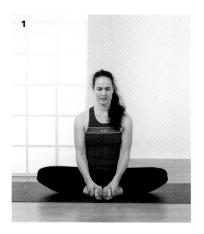

1

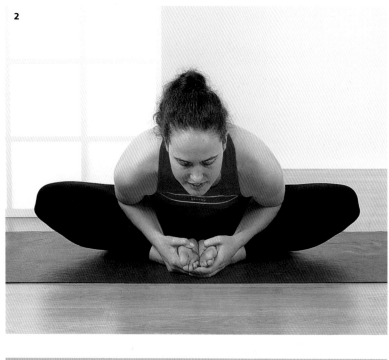

2

2 Press your feet together and take your knees to the floor. Keep your body straight and lift your lower back while holding onto your feet.
Breath: keep breathing evenly for 2–5 minutes.
Bend forward, using your elbows to keep your thighs pressed to the floor. Take your chest toward your feet and then rest your forehead on the floor.
Breath: keep breathing for eight or more breaths, then release the pose.

■ BEGINNER'S VERSION

If your hips and lower back are stiff, then your lower back will curve and your knees will stay lifted in this pose. So, practice this pose (see Steps 1 and 2) sitting on a block or folded blanket to lift your hips, and place a block under each knee. Also practice this pose against a wall for added support.

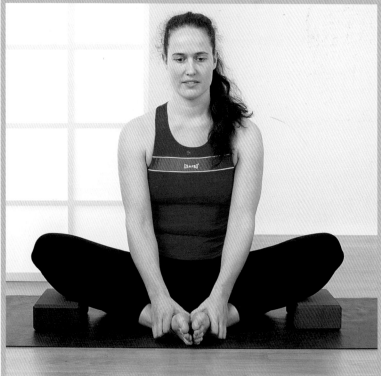

ūpavista konasana

Seated angle pose

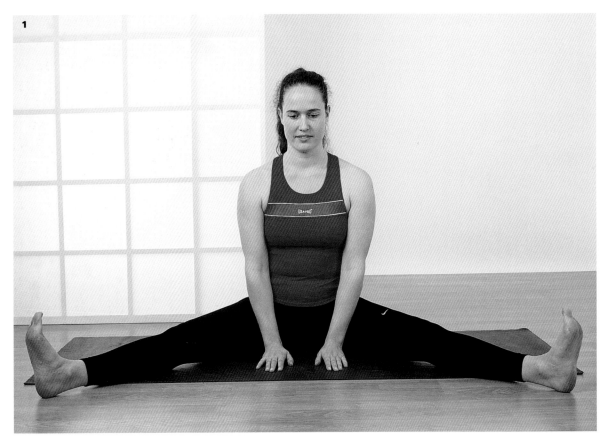

1

1 Sit upright in *dandasana* pose (see p.56).
Inhale: stretch both legs out to the side as wide as possible. Keep your knees and feet pointing upward. Press your thighs into the floor and push into your heels. Place your palms on the floor in front of you with your fingers spaced apart and facing forward.

2 Exhale: walk your fingers forward, taking your elbows to the floor. Keep your back flat and your thighs and sit bones pressing into the floor.
Breath: rest in the pose for a few breaths.

3 Inhale: straighten your arms out to the sides and take hold of your feet, keeping your chest lifted.
Exhale: pull on your feet and bend your chest toward the floor. Rest your chin on the floor. Keep your legs straight; do not roll them.
Breath: keep breathing evenly for eight or more breaths.
Inhale: come up, then **exhale** as you release the pose.

■ BEGINNER'S VERSION

The lower back has a tendency to sag or roll under in this pose. So, as a beginner, place a block or folded blanket under your buttocks in Step 1 to prevent sagging. Only bend as far forward as comfortable with a flat back.

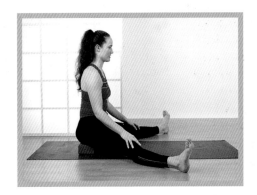

2

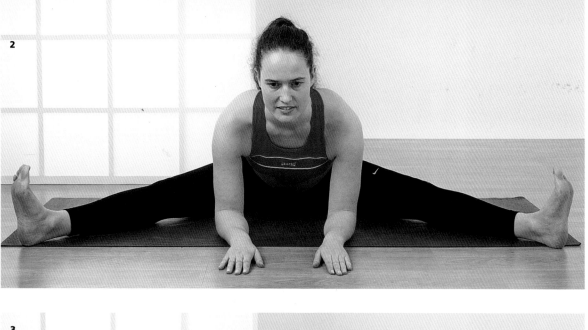

3

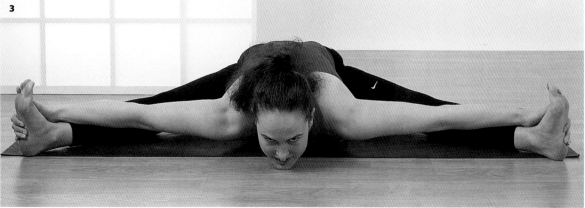

pārsva ūpavista konasana

Seated angle side stretch

Sit as in step 1 of *upavista konasana* (see opposite).

Exhale: bend sideways, extending over your right leg and take your right elbow to the floor. Rotate your arm and clasp your right foot, curling your fingers around the sole of your foot.

Inhale, then **exhale:** stretch your left arm by your ear to take hold of the outer edge of your right foot. Extend your body and rotate your chest to look up. Keep your left buttock pressing into the floor and stretch up from the waist.

Breath: keep breathing evenly for eight or more breaths.

Inhale: come up, then repeat on the other side.

CHAPTER 4

Twists and **Balancing** Poses

Twisting poses improve the lateral flexibility of your spine and they purify the spinal nerves. Twists are particularly helpful in relieving any stiffness in your back, neck, and shoulders. The squeezing motion of the spinal twists wrings out impurities held in the liver, kidneys and other organs of the abdomen and pelvis. When the twist is released a fresh supply of oxygenated blood flushes through your system and helps to wake up the digestive system and tone the lower organs.

Balancing poses focus and concentrate the mind, bringing you serenity and stillness. They strengthen the wrists and help to develop agility, grace and poise.

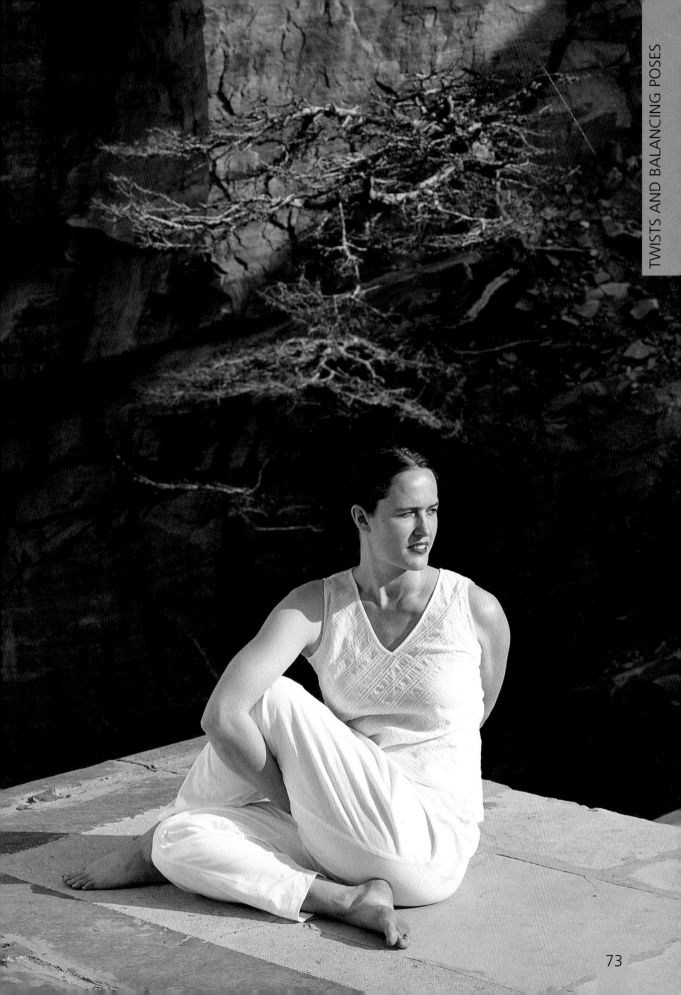

Twists *bharadvajasana*

Twisting on a chair

A gentle method for easing the body into twist asanas is to start by doing them on a chair.

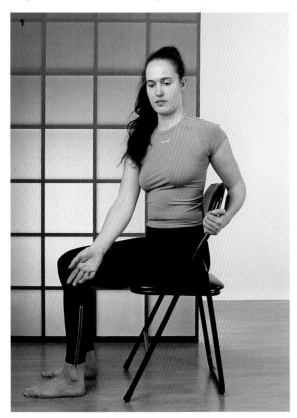

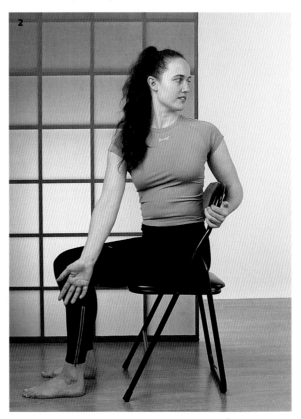

1 Sit on a chair with your feet and knees a hip width apart.
Inhale: place your feet firmly on the floor and keep your hips parallel.
Exhale: begin to rotate to the left to take hold of the side of the chair with your left hand. Place your right wrist on the outside of your left knee with the palm facing out.
Breath: keep breathing evenly.

2 Inhale, then **exhale:** increase the twist by pressing your right wrist against your left knee, using it as a lever, and pull against the chair with your left hand. Twist from the base of your spine, turning in your hips, waist, chest and finally your shoulders. Keep your neck and shoulders relaxed. Turn your head to look over your left shoulder.
Breath: keep breathing evenly for eight breaths.
Inhale: come back to center, exhale, and repeat on the other side.

WORKING WITH PROPS

■ Using props makes difficult asanas possible for all yoga students. They build the confidence and experience necessary to attempt complicated poses.

■ Any object can be used as a prop—a chair, stool, or a wall—as long as it helps you to experience the asana in a relaxed way. Be creative, but if you are using furniture make sure that it is stable and can bear your weight.

ardha matsyendrasana

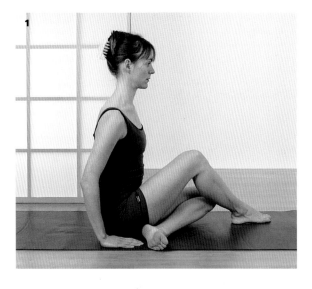

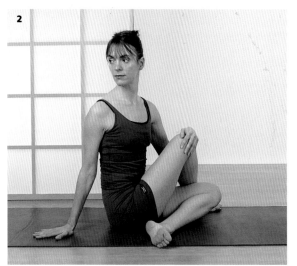

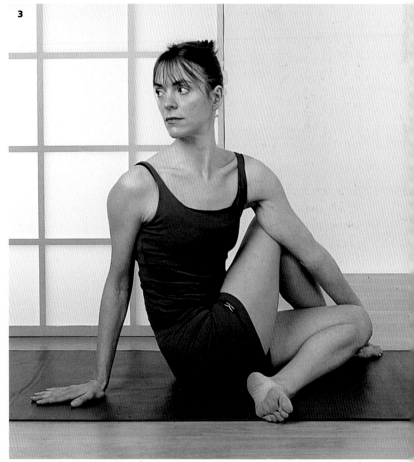

1 Sit upright in *dandasana* pose (see p.56). Bend your knees and place the soles of your feet on the floor 1½ ft/ 45 cm from your buttocks. Pass your left leg under the right, so that your knee is in front of your body with your left heel in line with your right hip.

2 **Inhale:** place your right foot on the outside of your left knee, with the sole flat on the floor. Lift up your torso and begin to twist toward your right leg, placing your right hand on the floor behind and looking over your right shoulder. Put your left hand on your right leg.

3 **Exhale:** hook your upper left arm over your right knee and twist more deeply. Move your left hand down to hold the sole of your right foot. Twist up from your spine, turning in your hips, waist, chest, and shoulders. Relax your shoulders and stay looking over your right shoulder.
Breath: keep breathing evenly for eight or more breaths.
Inhale: turn back to the center, **exhale,** and repeat on the other side.

marichyasana iii

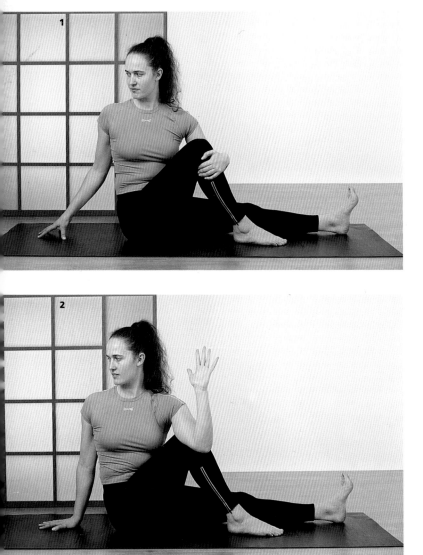

1 Sit upright in *dandasana* pose (see p.56). Bend your right knee and place your foot in line with your left knee.
Inhale: lift up and turn toward your bent leg, placing your right hand on the floor behind. Clasp your left hand around your left knee, pressing into the floor with your thigh and extending into your left heel.

2 Exhale: increase the twist and take your left arm to the outside of your right knee so that your palm faces the front. Turn your head to look over your right shoulder.
Breath: keep breathing evenly.

3 Inhale, then **exhale:** thread your left arm through the space in your bent leg. Wrap your right arm around your back to take hold of your right wrist with your left hand (see inset). Twist up from the base of the spine turning in the hips, waist, chest, and shoulders.
Breath: keep breathing evenly for eight or more breaths.
Inhale: turn back to the center, **exhale,** and repeat on the other side. If you find it difficult to twist, stay in Step 2.

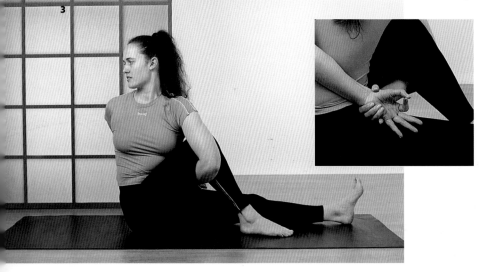

bharadvajasana ii

1 Sit upright in *dandasana* pose (see p.56).
Inhale: bend your left leg and take it back so that your foot is in line with your left hip. Use your thumb to pull your calf muscle out to the side, as in Step 1 of *triang mukhaikapada paschimottanasana* (see p.60). Bend your right leg and bring it into half lotus position by placing your foot on top of your left thigh close to the groin, with your right knee down.

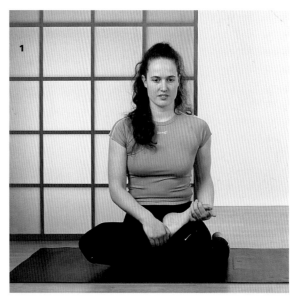

2 **Exhale:** turn your torso to the right. Wrap your right arm behind your back and take hold of your right foot. Place your left wrist on the outside of your right knee, using it as a lever to increase the twist. Turn your head to look over your right shoulder. Relax your shoulders.
Breath: keep breathing evenly for eight or more breaths.
Inhale: turn back to the center, exhale, and repeat on other side.

BENEFITS

- This lateral movement refreshes the spine by supplying blood to the nerves.
- The heel massages the intestines and helps eliminate any toxins.

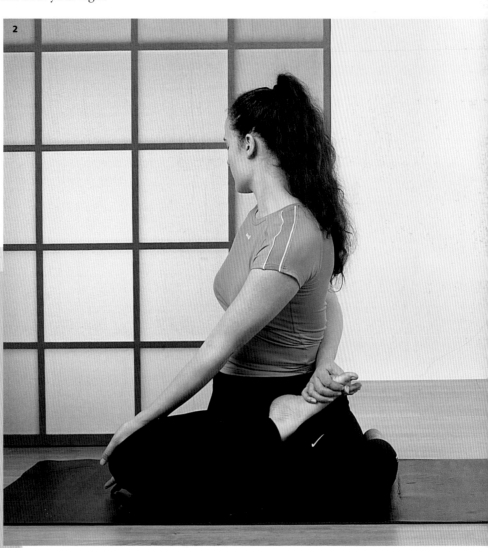

pasasana

Bound pose

Pasasana combines both balance and twisting movements.

1 Inhale: stand upright in *tadasana* pose (see p.38), then squat down.
Exhale: turn your torso to the right and place your right hand on the floor behind your right hip. Bend your left arm and take your elbow to the outside of your left knee with your forearm pointing up and your palm facing forward.

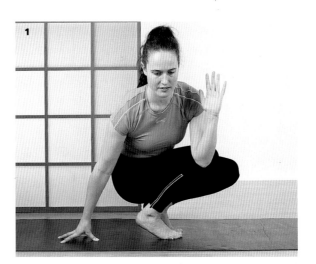

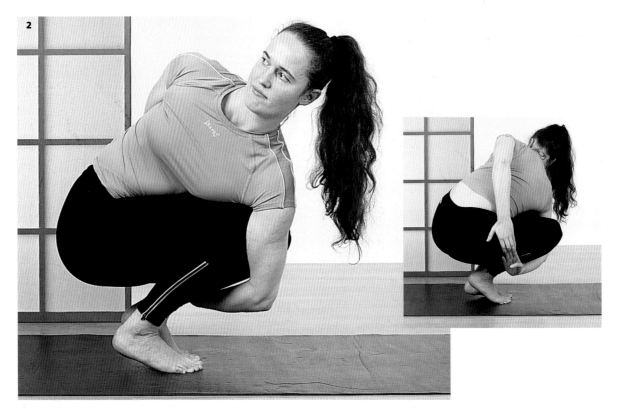

2 Press your left arm against your right leg to rotate your body and turn your chest.
Breath: keep breathing evenly.
Inhale, and as you **exhale:** lean closer toward your bent legs, sliding your left armpit down the outside of your right knee. Wrap your left arm back and around your bent knees to bind your legs, taking your left hand to the outside of your left shin. Lift your right shoulder back and take your right arm behind your back to catch hold of your left hand (see inset) with your fingertips, then move your hands closer to increase the turn. Look over your right shoulder while working your heels toward the floor. If necessary, put a folded blanket under your heels for support.
Breath: breathe evenly for eight or more breaths.
Inhale: turn back to the center, **exhale**, and repeat on the other side.

parsva bakasana

Side crow pose

1 Stand upright in *tadasana* pose (see p.38), then come into a squatting position facing the front. Twist to the left and place your hands down on the floor, a hip-width apart, to the outside of your left knee and spread out your fingers. Focus your eyes on a point in front of you.

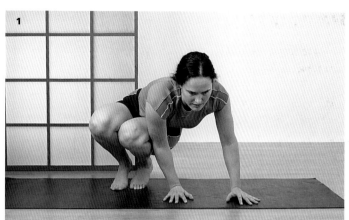

2 Bend your elbows back and balance your knees on top of your right forearm. Slowly shift your weight forward and slightly to the left to keep some weight on this side. Slowly raise your feet out to the right side, keeping your legs together.

Breath: keep breathing evenly for eight or more breaths, then release the pose.

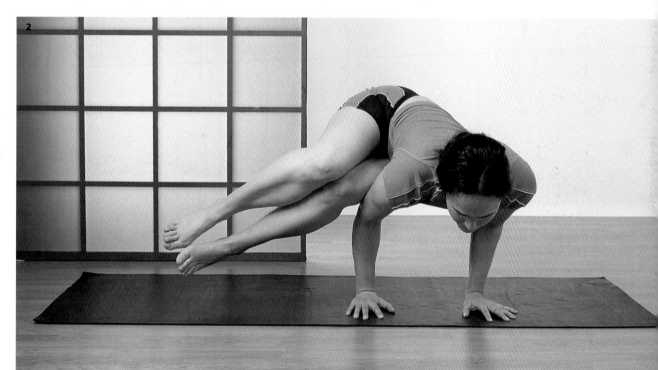

BENEFITS

■ *Bakasana* and *parsva bakasana* greatly develop your powers of concentration, preparing your mind for the one-pointed concentration that is needed for deep meditation.

■ The postures promote lightness in the body and a feeling of inner poise.

■ They strengthen the arms and wrists and revitalize the nerves of the arms, helping conditions such as tendonitis.

83

CHAPTER 5

Reclining and Backbending Poses

Reclining poses are very restful, as they allow your body to be supported by the earth. They relieve compression in the spine, aiding the nervous system. They also help to open the groin and lubricate the joints. The poses are calming, building energy, and developing the flexibility that is necessary for more strenuous poses.

Backbending poses strengthen the muscles in the back, stretch the spine, and stimulate the *sushumna nadi* (an important energy channel). They expand the chest, opening the heart center, giving energy, courage, and mental clarity. Practicing these asanas can help to overcome depression. They also increase the space between the organs, removing toxins and allowing vital nutrients and blood to flow freely. After backbending, release the spine gently in the opposite direction by coming into child's pose (see p.101).

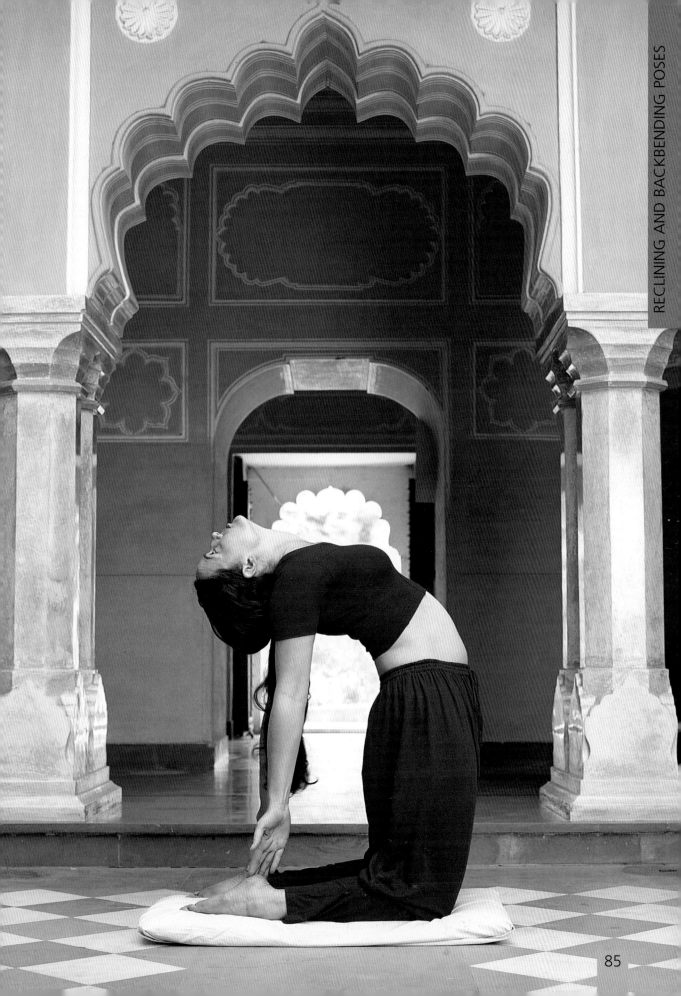

supta padangusthasana

Lying thumb to foot pose

1 **Inhale:** lie on your back with your legs together and feet flexed. Bend your left leg and grasp your big toe with your thumb, index and middle finger of your left hand. Lift up and straighten your left leg, stretching into your heel. Keep your left shoulder down, your hips level and right leg strong by pushing down with your right thigh. Take your right arm to the side, palm down.

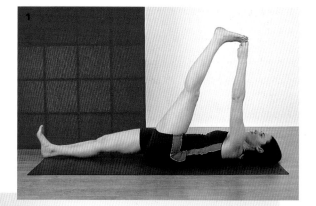

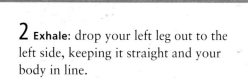

2 **Exhale:** drop your left leg out to the left side, keeping it straight and your body in line.
Breath: keep breathing evenly for eight or more breaths.
Inhale: come back to the center, **exhale**, release the leg, and then repeat on the other side.

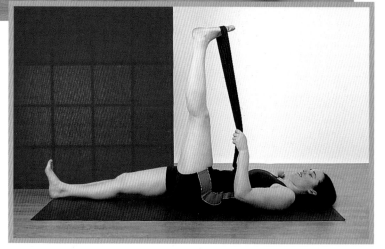

■ **BEGINNER'S VERSION**
If you are finding it difficult to reach your big toe and straighten your leg with your shoulder down, then place a belt around the ball of your left foot in Step 1. Hold the belt firmly and take your leg out to the side.

parivartanasana

Lying side stretch

1 Lie on your back with your body in a straight line. Bend both knees up toward your chest. Stretch your arms out to the sides, placing your palms face down on the floor. Relax your face.

Breath: keep breathing evenly.

2 Inhale, then as you **exhale:** drop your knees over to the left side, rotating from the waist. Keep your right shoulder moving down toward the floor. Turn your head to look over to your right side. Relax your neck and release your back.

Breath: keep breathing evenly for eight or more breaths.

Inhale: bring your legs to the center, **exhale** and repeat on the other side.

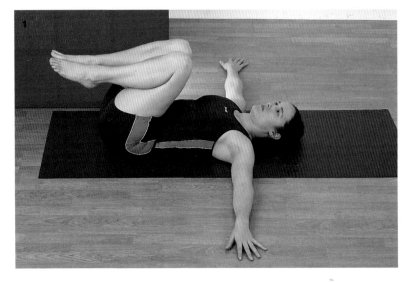

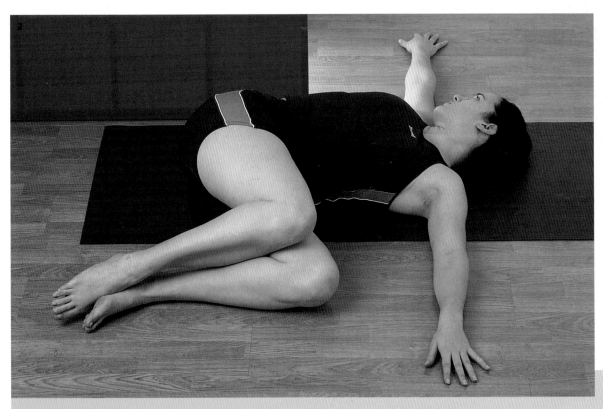

BENEFITS

■ This pose is very good for relieving back pain as it helps to release the muscles that are tensing in the lower back.

supta
virasana

Hero pose

1 From kneeling, lift your buttocks up so that you balance on your knees. Keep them together and move your feet a little wider than a hip-width apart, with your toes pointing backward. Slowly sit back down between your feet, easing your calf muscles out to the sides with your thumbs (see *triang mukhaikapada paschimottanasana* pp.60–61). Sit up straight, lifting up from the sit bones (near your hip bones).

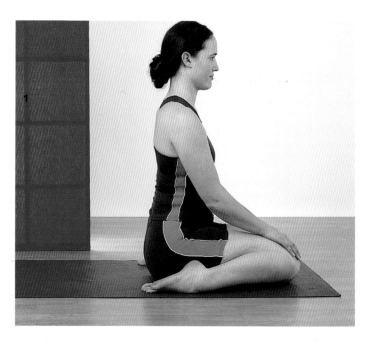

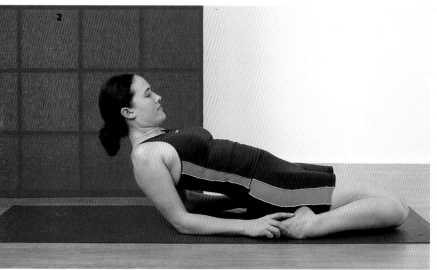

2 **Inhale,** and as you **exhale:** gently lower yourself back onto your elbows and tuck your tailbone under. Feel the stretch through your thighs and groin. **Breath:** keep breathing evenly throughout.

3 **Inhale,** and as you **exhale:** continue the stretch by taking your back and head down to the ground. Tuck your chin in slightly. Stretch your arms over your head and take hold of your elbows. Stretch up from your waist to the elbows, opening out from the armpits, and down from the waist toward your kneecaps. Keep your body evenly extended. There should be no knee pain as the stretch is through the front of the body. **Breath:** keep breathing evenly for eight or more breaths. **Inhale:** slowly come up, then gently **exhale.**

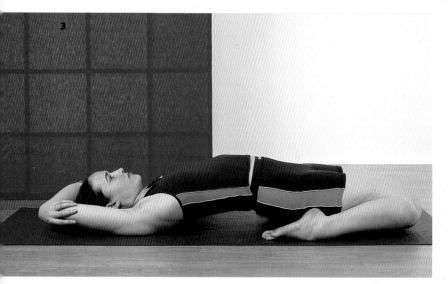

adho mukha svanasana

Downward facing dog pose

Lie on your stomach. Place your palms on the floor just below your shoulders, with fingers pointing forward. Keep your feet a hip-width apart and tuck your toes under. Push up onto your knees.

Inhale, and then as you **exhale:** push into your palms and raise your buttocks up and back, flattening your back into a triangle. Keep your hips high and stretch your heels down, opening the backs of the knees. Point your head toward the floor.

Breath: keep breathing evenly for eight or more breaths, then release the pose.

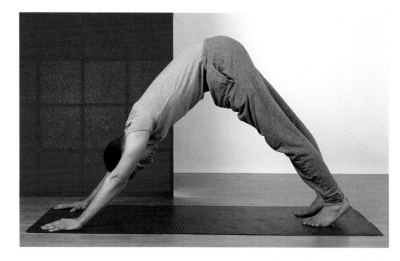

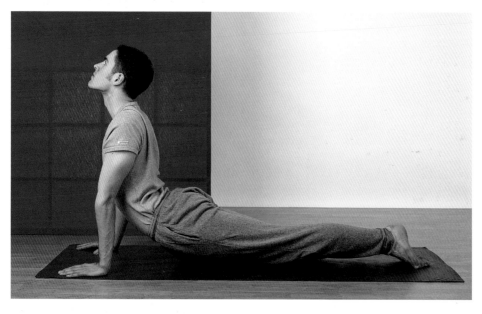

ūrdhva mukha svanasana

Upward facing dog pose

Lie down on your stomach. Place your palms on the floor just below your shoulders, with your fingers pointing forward. Keep your feet a hip-width apart and point your toes. Lift your head and chest and arch your upper back.

Inhale: push into your palms and straighten your arms. Tighten your leg muscles and lift your legs a few inches from the floor to balance on your toes.

Exhale: push your chest forward and up between your arms, pulling your legs forward, and look up toward the ceiling. Relax your shoulders down.

Breath: keep breathing evenly eight or more breaths, then release the pose.

bhujangasana

Cobra pose

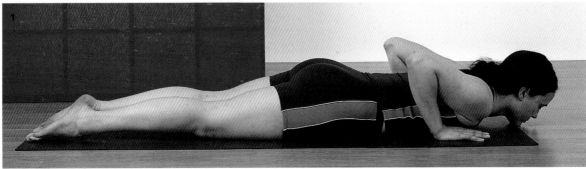

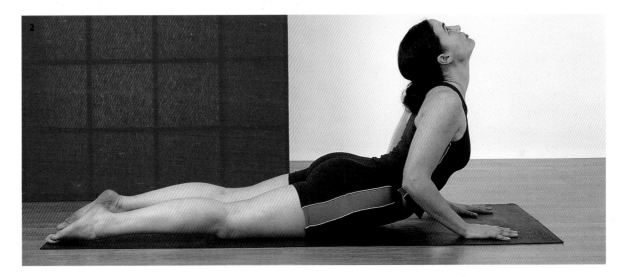

1 **Inhale:** lie flat on your stomach. Bring your feet and legs together and place your palms under your shoulders beside your ribcage. Place your forehead and then your chin on the floor. Feel the extension through the spine from the tailbone to the crown of your head.

2 **Exhale:** without pressing into your hands, raise your head and chest. Roll your shoulders down and open your chest. Press into your palms, lengthening your spine vertebra by vertebra, bringing your chest forward. Keep your elbows by your body. Stretch up your chin, looking toward the ceiling.
Breath: keep breathing evenly for eight or more breaths, then release the pose.

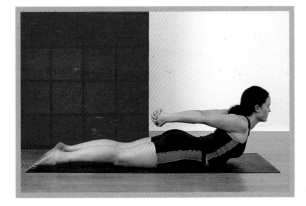

■ BEGINNER'S VERSION

As a beginner, you need to strengthen your back muscles without overextending your spine. Lie on your stomach as in Step 1, and take your feet a hip-width apart. Place your forehead and then chin on the floor. Clasp your hands behind your back and stretch toward your feet, lifting your head and chest.
Breath: keep breathing evenly for eight or more breaths, then release the pose.

Salabhasana

Locust pose

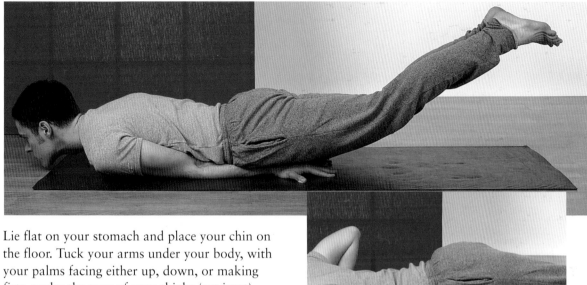

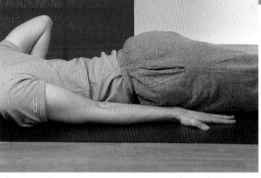

Lie flat on your stomach and place your chin on the floor. Tuck your arms under your body, with your palms facing either up, down, or making fists, under the tops of your thighs (see inset). Move your elbows as close together as possible.
Inhale: stretch your legs back and up.
Exhale: keeping your legs together and straight.
Breath: keep breathing evenly for eight breaths or more, then release the pose.

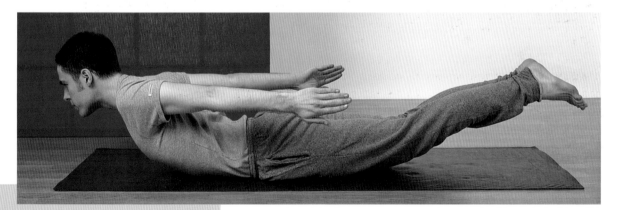

BENEFITS

■ *Salabhasana* and its variation (I) strengthen the muscles of your lower back, pelvis, and abdomen.

■ The poses tone the intestines and help to relieve constipation.

Locust pose I

Lie flat on your stomach. Place your chin on the floor and bring your feet together, with your arms stretching out behind your body. Tuck your tailbone under, pressing your pubic bone into the ground.
Inhale: lift your head, chest and legs as high as possible.
Exhale: press your shoulder blades into your back and stretch your arms toward your feet. Keep your feet and legs together. Do not strain into your lower back.
Breath: keep breathing evenly for eight or more breaths, then release the pose.

dhanurasana

Bow pose

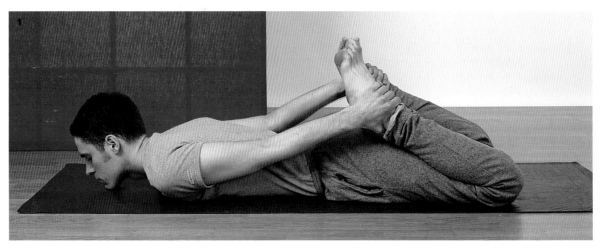

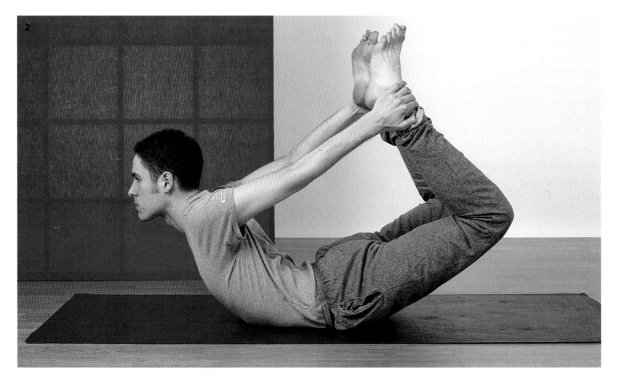

1 Lie flat on your stomach and rest your forehead on the floor. Keep your feet a hip-width apart, bend your knees, and take your heels toward your buttocks. Stretch your arms back and take hold of the outside of your ankles. Tuck your tailbone under and put your chin on the floor.
Breath: keep breathing evenly.

2 Inhale: raise your legs up and back. Keep pulling up with your legs. Allow the force of your legs to lift your head and chest up as high as possible to arch your back, but let your spine remain passive. Keep your arms straight, relax your shoulders and balance on your abdomen.
Exhale: raise your chin and try to look up toward the ceiling.
Breath: keep breathing evenly for eight or more breaths, then release the pose.

ūstrasana

Camel pose

1 Kneel with your thighs and buttocks lifted, bringing your knees a hip-width apart. Place your hands on your waist and extend your spine up. Lean back and begin to lift your sternum up toward the ceiling.

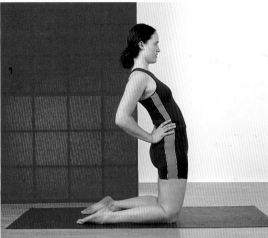

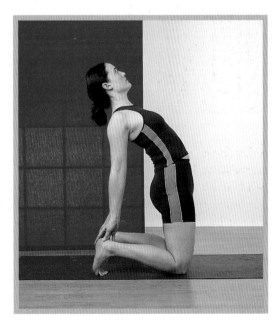

2 **Inhale:** keeping your hips in line with your knees and your tailbone tucked under, arch your back. Move your shoulder blades down and into your upper back to open your chest.

Exhale: stretch evenly along your spine. Reach your arms down and place your hands on your heels. Keep your shins pressing into the floor. Extend your neck and look back.

Breath: keep breathing evenly eight or more times, then release the pose.

■ BEGINNER'S VERSION

Developing flexibility in the spine takes time and effort for a beginner, and reaching the heels is difficult. To work in the pose come up onto your toes in Step 2 to make it easier to reach your heels. Keep your head lifted to avoid constricting the back of your neck.

Chakrasana

Wheel pose

1 Lie flat on your back. Bend your legs and place your feet on the floor close to your buttocks. Stretch your arms toward your feet and hold the backs of your ankles. Tuck your tailbone under.
Breath: keep breathing evenly.

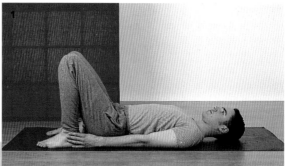

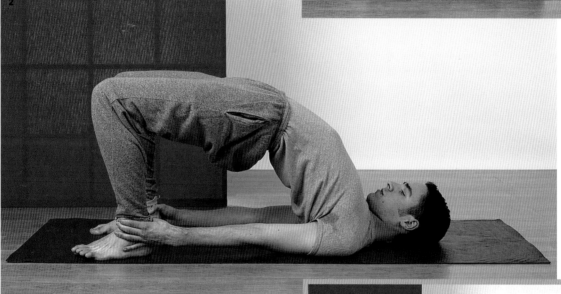

2 **Inhale,** then as you **exhale:** push into your heels and raise your pelvis up. Roll onto the tops of your shoulders and lift your chest. Tuck your chin in, stretching the back of your neck. Keep your thighs strong and your knees in line with your heels.
Breath: keep breathing evenly for eight or more breaths, then release the pose gently, placing one vertebra at a time back down onto the floor.

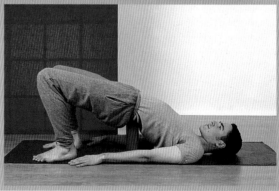

BENEFITS

- *Chakrasana* is a useful pose for preparing for both *urdhva dhanurasana* (see p.95) and *sarvangasana* (see pp.104–106).
- The pose opens the shoulders and the hip joints and develops flexibility in the spine.
- It is especially useful for women as it helps to regulate the menstrual cycle.

■ BEGINNER'S VERSION
This is a gentle and passive way to practice this pose as a beginner to develop flexibility in the spine. Lift your hips as in Step 2 and place a block underneath your sacrum, either lengthways or vertically, depending on how high your hips are lifted, to support your lower back.
Breath: relax and breathe normally for eight or more breaths.

ūrdhva dhanurasana

Upward bow pose

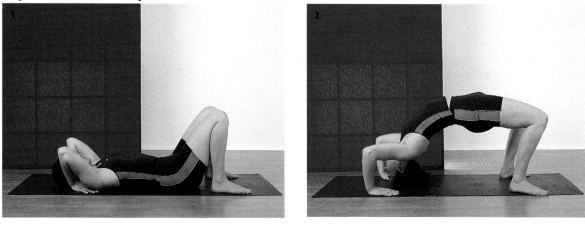

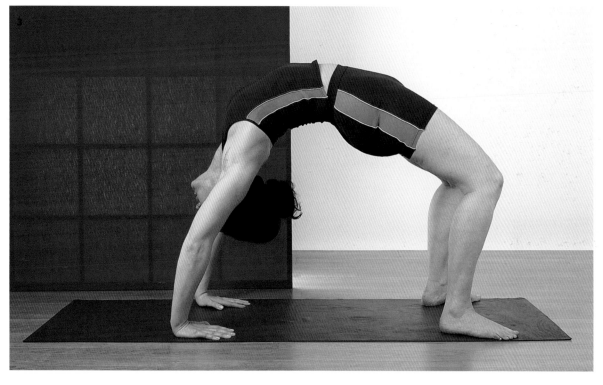

1 Lie on your back. Bend your legs and place your feet on the floor close to your buttocks. Bend your elbows and place your palms flat down on the floor underneath your shoulders.
Breath: keep breathing evenly.

2 Inhale, then as you **exhale:** push into your hands and feet, raise your pelvis, and place the crown of your head on the floor.
Breath: keep breathing evenly.

3 Inhale, then as you **exhale:** push into your palms, lift your navel and raise your hips as high as possible. Tuck your tailbone under. Straighten your arms and keep lifting your thighs. Look down toward the floor.
Breath: breathe evenly for eight or more breaths, then release the pose.

CHAPTER 6

Inversion
Poses

According to the yoga text, head and shoulder stands are the king and queen of asanas. Inverted poses have a tremendous effect on the body and mind. They help to regulate the endocrine system, especially the pineal, pituitary, thyroid, and parathyroid glands in the head and neck. These glands regulate the emotional and metabolic processes of the body by secreting hormones into the bloodstream. Regularly practicing the inverted asanas reduces stress, anxiety, and nervous energy, even affecting our thought processes.

The inversion pose reverses the gravitational orientation of the body, sending a rich supply of blood to the brain, which refreshes the nerve cells and rests the heart. Turning our world upside down can help us to gain a new perspective on life, and throw out any limiting modes of behavior. After inversions, to avoid dizziness as you come upright, always release into child's pose (see p.101).

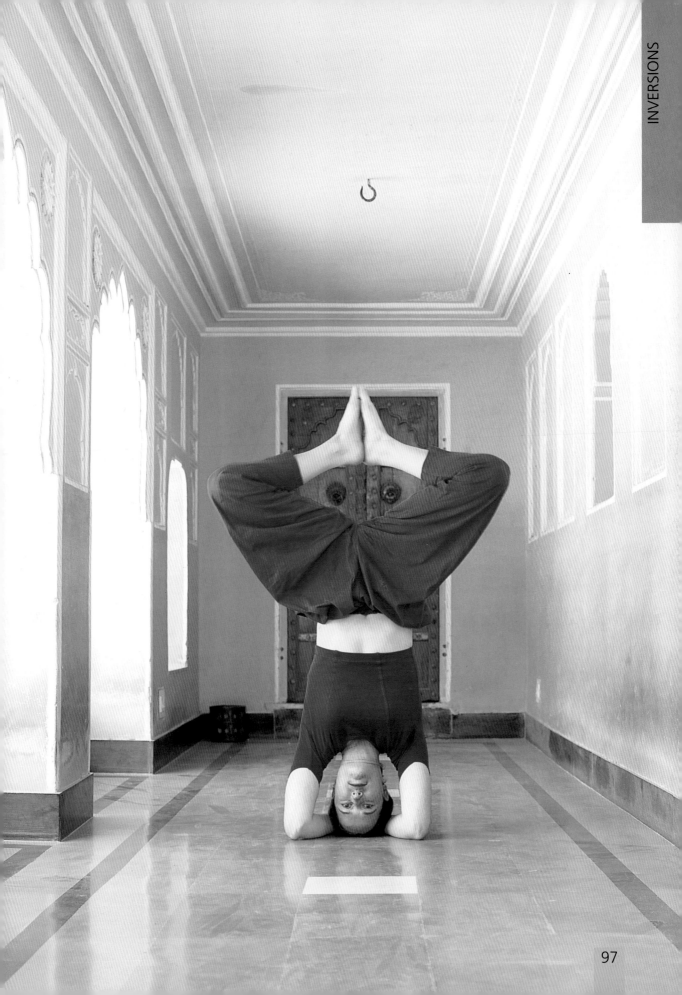

adho mukha vrkasana

Face down tree pose

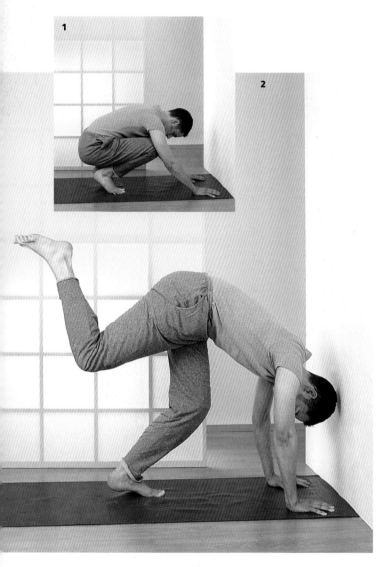

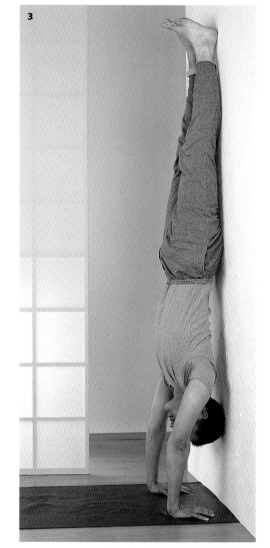

1 Squat down and place your hands, palms down and a shoulder-width apart, on the mat in front of you about 2–3 in/50–76 mm from the wall.

2 Raise your hips, straighten your arms and begin to bring your body weight into your hands. Keep the crown of your head pointing toward the floor. **Inhale,** then as you **exhale:** kick your right leg up toward the wall followed by your left, so that you are balancing against the wall.

3 Push up from your palms, straighten your elbows, and lift up your shoulders and chest. Tuck your tailbone in to reduce the arch in your back. Bring your feet together, make your legs strong, and extend your heels upward.
Breath: keep breathing evenly for eight or more breaths. Come down by dropping one leg toward the floor. Return to a squatting position for a few minutes before standing.

pinca mayurasana

Fan-tailed peacock pose

1

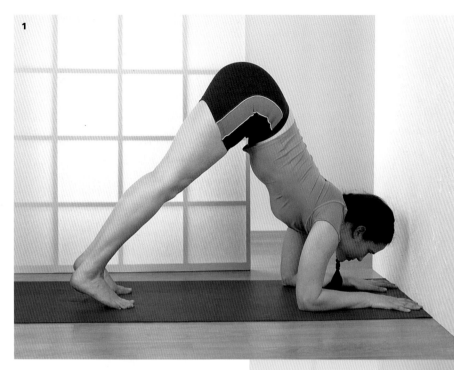

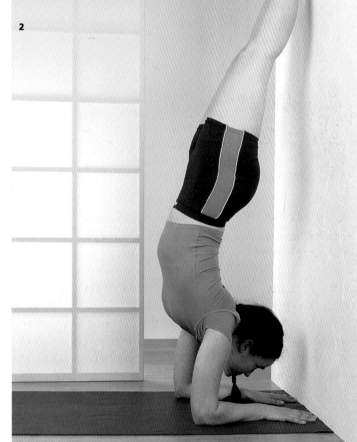

1 **Inhale:** from a kneeling position, place your forearms on the floor with your palms flat on the mat and your fingertips close to the wall. Keep your elbows a shoulder-width apart. Straighten your legs, raise your hips, and look forward between your hands. Start to shift your body weight into your elbows.

2 **Exhale:** kick your right leg up toward the wall, followed by your left leg. Bring your feet and legs together to rest your heels against the wall, keeping your thigh muscles strong. Push into the floor with your forearms and try to balance on your elbows. Lift your shoulders and look forward.
Breath: keep breathing evenly for eight or more breaths. Come down by dropping one leg toward the floor. Return to a squatting position for a few minutes before standing.

2

sirsasana

Dolphin pose
(Preparing for headstand)

Practicing the dolphin pose develops strength in your shoulders, upper back, and chest in preparation for a headstand.

1 From a kneeling position, bend forward, place your forearms on the floor, and clasp your fingers with the heel of your hands on the floor. Keep your elbows a shoulder-width apart. Press with your arms, straighten your legs, and raise your hips as in downward facing dog (see p.89).
Inhale: slowly lower your body down in front of your hands.

2 Exhale: pressing into your forearms, lift your body up, forward, and over your hands, taking your chin down toward the floor.
Repeat Steps 1 and 2 eight or more times. Gradually build up the number of repetitions over time.

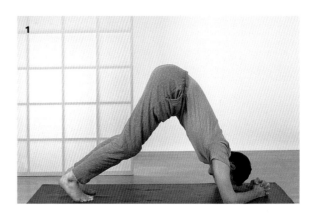

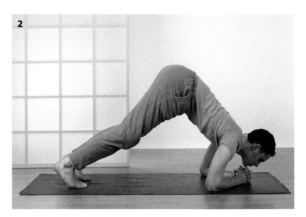

Headstand for beginners

It is helpful for beginners to practice a headstand against a wall to prevent rolling backward.

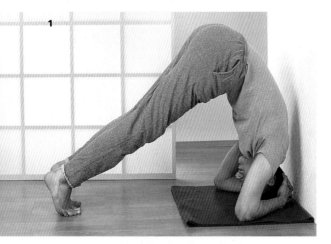

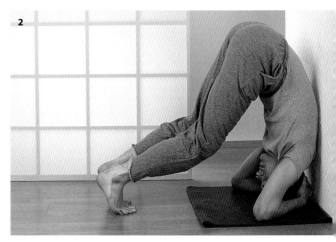

1 From kneeling, place your elbows on the mat underneath your shoulders. Clasp your fingers and put your hands on the floor, with your thumb pointing up, so that your arms form an equilateral triangle. Place the crown of your head on the floor in front of your hands. Straighten your legs.
Breath: keep breathing evenly.

2 Begin to walk your feet forward, and raise your hips until they are in line with your head. Press your forearms down and distribute the weight of your body between your arms and head.
Breath: keep breathing evenly.

3 Bend your knees in toward your chest and raise your feet off the floor.
Inhale, then as you **exhale**: lift your knees, placing the soles of your feet on the wall.
Breath: keep breathing evenly.

4 Extend your legs up the wall. Keep raising up from your forearms, lift your shoulders, and tuck your tailbone under. The weight of your body should be symmetrically balanced. Relax your face and allow gravity to do the work.
Breath: keep breathing evenly for eight or more breaths. Come down by dropping one leg toward the floor. Return to a squatting position for a few minutes before standing.

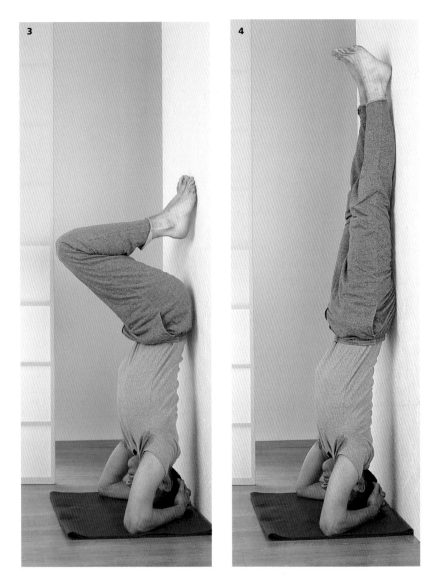

Child's pose

It is important not to jump up after an inversion as the blood rushes from the head and can cause dizziness. Child's pose is the perfect posture between inversions.

From a kneeling position, bend forward and place your forehead on the floor in front of your knees. Move your arms back by your body, so that your hands line up with your feet. Relax your shoulders and release your buttocks toward your heels.
Breath: breathe slowly and quietly for as long as necessary.

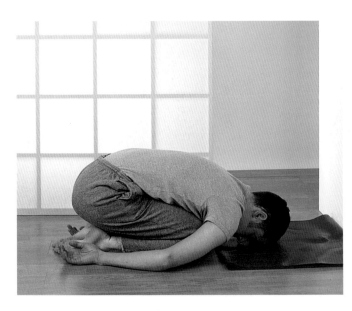

sirsasana

Headstand

▶ After practicing the beginner's headstand (see pp.100–101), you can move away from the wall. To do a freestanding headstand, go up in the normal way but move a couple of inches from the wall, and then keep moving further away. Once you've developed the poise necessary to practice the headstand in the center of the room, and can stay in it for 5–10 minutes, go on to the variations.

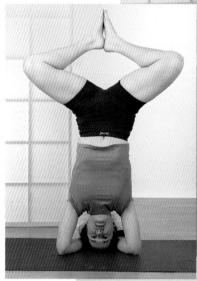

Headstand with feet together

Come into *sirsasana* (see above).
▶ **Inhale**, then as you **exhale:** bend your knees out to the sides and bring your soles of your feet together with the toes pointing up. Draw your feet as close to your groin as possible and maintain a steady balance.
Breath: keep breathing evenly for eight or more breaths. Come down by dropping one leg toward the floor. Return to a squatting position for a few minutes before standing, or do another variation.

WARNING
Do not attempt a headstand if you have high blood pressure, glaucoma, whiplash, are menstruating or are over four months pregnant.

Headstand with legs apart

▶ Come into *sirsasana* (see above).
Inhale, then as you **exhale:** open your legs out to the side as wide as possible. Stretch along the inside of your legs, pushing out toward the heels. Try to maintain a steady balance.
Breath: keep breathing evenly for eight or more breaths. Come down by dropping one leg toward the floor. Return to a squatting position for a few minutes before standing, or do another variation.

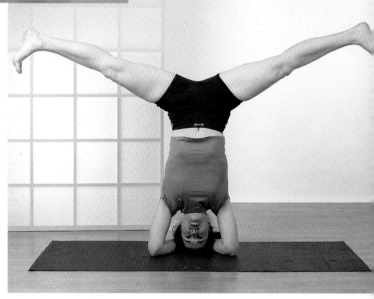

Headstand with legs at right angle to the body

▼ Come into *sirsasana* (see left). Bring your legs together, flex your feet and strengthen your thighs. **Inhale,** then as you **exhale:** slowly lower your legs, using your abdominal muscles until they are at a right angle. Lift your body up toward your sit bones (near your hip bones), and try to maintain a steady balance.

Breath: keep breathing evenly for eight breaths. **Inhale,** then as you **exhale:** lift your legs back up until they are vertical. Come down by dropping one leg toward the floor. Return to a squatting position for a few minutes before standing, or do another variation.

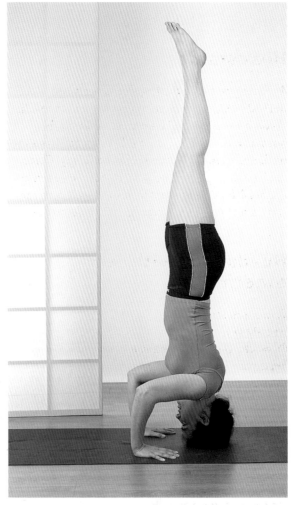

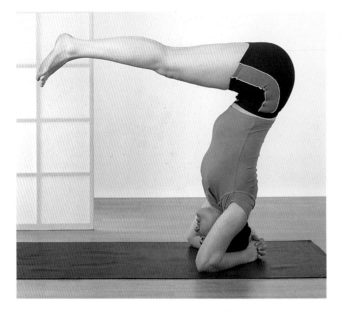

BENEFITS

■ *Sirsasana* rejuvenates your brain, improves your memory and tones your nervous system.

■ It has a positive effect on your endocrine glands in the head and neck.

■ The pose also improves asthma and other ailments of the lungs.

Headstand I

▲ Only attempt this asana once you are comfortable in *sirsasana* and the variations. It expands your concentration and balance before meditation.

From a kneeling position, place your palms with fingers spread on the mat in line with your shoulders. Place your head on the floor in between and just in front of your fingers until your arms form a right angle. Straighten your legs, raise your hips, and walk your feet forward until your hips line up with your head.

Inhale, then as you **exhale:** bend your knees in toward your chest. Lift your feet off the floor and raise your legs until they are vertical. Keep the weight on your head with your hands as stabilizers. **Breath:** keep breathing evenly for eight or more breaths. Come down by dropping one leg toward the floor. Return to a squatting position for a few minutes before standing.

ṣaʀvaṇgaṣaṇa

Shoulder stand

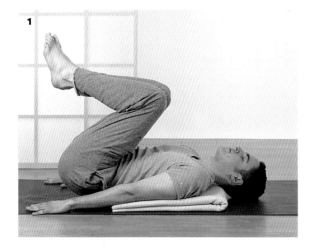

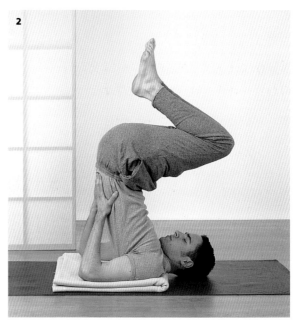

Sarvangasana is the queen of asanas. It helps to activate the thyroid and parathyroid glands, benefiting circulation, digestion and breathing. The variations also tone the body and regulate bowel function.

1 Put a folded blanket on the mat. Lie on your back with your shoulders in line with the edge of the blanket and your head on the floor. Tuck your chin in slightly and lengthen the back of your neck. Place your hands palms down beside you.
Inhale, then as you **exhale:** bend your knees. Push into your palms and raise your legs over your head.

2 Bend your arms and place your hands in the middle of your back for support, tucking in your elbows. Bring your torso to a vertical position, moving your chest toward your chin with your knees bent.

3 Lift your legs straight up in line with your torso. Also keep your shoulders, hips, and ankles in line. Tuck your tailbone under, lengthen your spine and relax your facial muscles.
Breath: breathe quietly for about a minute.
To come down, bend your knees and put your hands on the floor behind you, palms down. Slowly roll out of the pose, head down, placing one vertebra at a time on the floor. Release your legs onto the floor and relax, or do the variations.

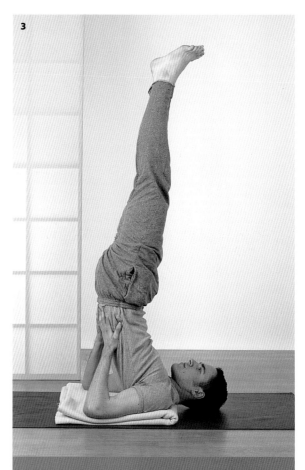

WARNING
Do not practice a shoulder stand if you have a neck injury, high blood pressure, are menstruating, or have a hernia. If you feel any pressure in your head, come out of the pose immediately.

Shoulder stand with one leg to the floor

▶ Come into *sarvangasana* (see opposite). Slowly take your left leg down toward the floor. Keep your right leg vertical and strong, stretching up into your right heel. Try to keep your hips level.

Breath: keep breathing evenly for about eight breaths, release and repeat on the other side.

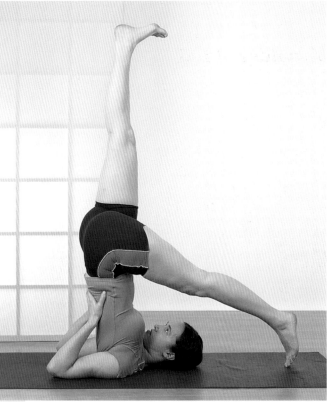

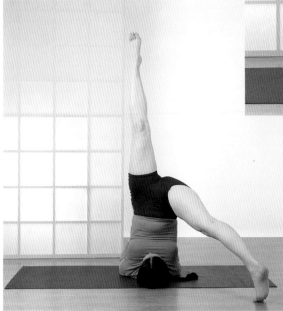

Shoulder stand with one leg to the side

◀ Come into *sarvangasana* (see opposite) with your feet together. Rotate your right leg so that the back of your heel lines up with your left instep. Then slowly take your right foot out to the side until it touches the floor. Keep your hips level.

Breath: keep breathing evenly for about eight breaths, release and repeat on the other side.

Shoulder stand with both legs out to the side

◀ Come into *sarvangasana* (see opposite) with your feet together. Rotate your right leg in its socket so that the back of the heel lines up with your left instep. Now slowly take your right foot out to the side. Then repeat with your left leg so that both feet are on the floor. Release your hands from behind your back and take hold of your feet.

Breath: keep breathing evenly for eight or more breaths, do another variation, or take a hand to support your back and lift the legs one at a time, then release as opposite.

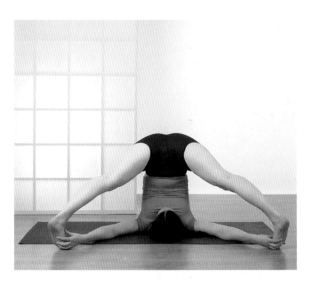

sarvangasana

Shoulder stand continued

Shoulder stand with both legs to one side

▶ Come into *sarvangasana* (see p.104).
Inhale, then as you exhale: slowly lower both your legs down to the floor. Move your right foot out to the side, then take your left leg to join the right. Keep your legs lifted and stretch into your heels.
Breath: keep breathing evenly for eight or more breaths. Walk your feet back to the center and then repeat on the other side.

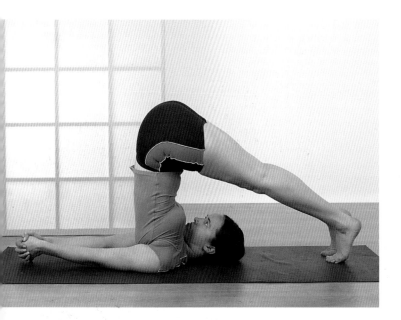

Shoulder stand with both legs down

◀ Come into *sarvangasana* (see p.104), keep both your legs together, and slowly lower them down to the floor behind your head using strong abdominal muscles. Place the tips of your toes on the mat behind your head. Your hips should be in line with your shoulders, with the backs of your thighs lifting toward the ceiling. Release your hands from your back, clasp your fingers, and stretch your arms away from your feet.
Breath: keep breathing evenly for eight or more breaths. Slowly roll out of the pose or move on to another variation.

Shoulder stand with knees by ears

▶ Come into *sarvangasana* (see p.104) then lower both your feet to the floor behind your head, and take your feet 1 ft/30 cm apart. Bend your knees and place them on the floor beside your ears, resting on your feet. Release your hands from behind your back and take them beside your calves to take hold of your feet.
Breath: keep breathing evenly for eight or more breaths. Slowly roll out of the pose or move on to another variation.

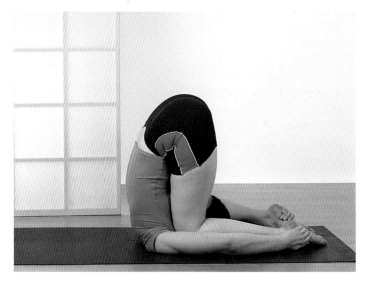

matsyasana

Fish pose

Fish pose should always be performed after a shoulder stand as it gives a reverse stretch to the neck.

Lie on your back. Bring your legs together and place the palms of your hands on the floor by your thighs. Without moving your elbows, sit up slightly to look at your feet. Lift your chest, tilt your pelvis forward, and arch your back, placing the crown of your head on the floor. Relax your shoulders toward the floor. Look up toward the third eye center in the middle of your forehead.

Breath: keep breathing evenly for about eight breaths. Release, and slowly lift out of the pose.

viparita karani

Legs up the wall

This is a restful pose that prepares you for deep relaxation.

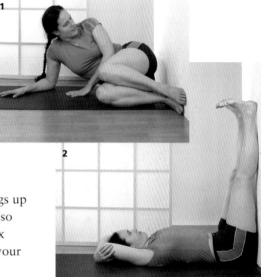

1 Sit in a sideways position and shift your buttocks close to the wall, with your left hip pointing upward.

2 Once your buttocks are in place, release the side of your torso to the floor, roll over onto your back, and lift your legs up the wall. If necessary, shift your buttocks closer to the wall so that the backs of both legs are in contact with the wall. Flex your feet and extend through the backs of your legs. Take your arms over your head and clasp the elbows.

Breath: relax for a few minutes breathing evenly.

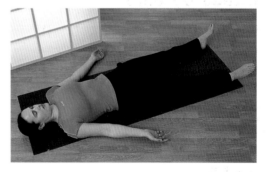

savasana

Relaxation pose

After yoga spend at least ten minutes in this pose to absorb the benefits and allow *prana* to flow freely.

Lie on your back. Place your feet a shoulder-width apart and relax your feet to the sides. Keep your hands a little way from your body with palms up. Slowly roll your head from side to side to release neck tension. Then release your body to the floor and breathe softly and gently. Mentally scan your body for tension areas. If you find any, then clench that body part and squeeze the tension out, then release it. Give yourself the time to let go.

CHAPTER 7

Pranayama and Meditation

Practicing the asanas tones and strengthens the physical body, the *annamaya kosha*, and purifies the nervous system. However, to work with the subtle aspect of our being—the mind—the higher practices of pranayama (breathing exercises) and meditation need to be performed. The breath and the mind are closely connected, for example; breathing is one of the involuntary functions of the body that can be directed and controlled by the mind. Pranayama acts as a bridge between the conscious and the subconscious and begins the process of drawing the mind away from external stimulus back toward its source, to a calm and quiet state. Once the mind is settled, then the practices of meditation can begin—these are collectively termed raja yoga. Raja yoga means the mastery of the mind and the senses. The joy of practicing yoga is that we are able to direct our energies in ways that are both positive for ourselves and others, and these can provide lasting contentment.

In this chapter are simple pranayama exercises, along with methods for preparating for meditation.

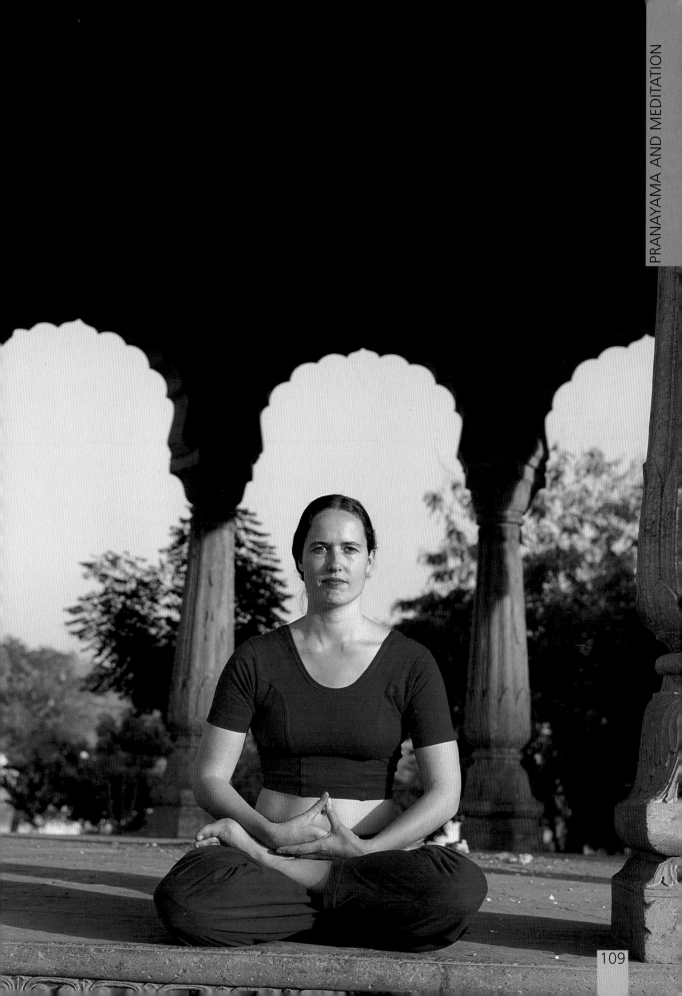

Pranayama

"When the breath wanders or is irregular, the mind is also unsteady, but when the breath is still so is the mind".

Hatha Yoga Pradipika ch. 2. v. 2

Pranayama literally means to control or expand *prana* through the subtle energy channels of the body. *Prana* is the life force or the vital energy that is said to be present in all forms of life. The Indian yogis have been quoted as saying that you can live without food for a few weeks, water for a few days, air for a few minutes, but not one second without *prana*—this is because *prana* animates and gives life to the body.

On a psychic level, the exercises of pranayama clear the subtle energy channels of the body, the *nadis*, allowing the energy to flow freely without blockages. *Prana*, within the inner channels, is intimately connected to thoughts. So when the breathing exercises are practiced, they set off sympathetic vibrations in the inner channels, which change the pattern of our thoughts, bringing us both peace and serenity.

A MIND LINK

Pranayama acts as a bridge between the conscious and unconscious areas of the mind, because breathing is an unconscious activity that can be influenced by the conscious mind. There is a direct correlation between the mind and the breath. The brain operates on a higher rate of metabolism than other organs, so it requires more oxygen to work efficiently. Our moods also affect our breathing, for example, when we are afraid, our rate of breathing becomes fast and shallow, but when we stop to take a deep breath, it slows down the heart rate and helps to relieve anxiety. On a physical level, breathing exercises purify the blood-stream. When we inhale, oxygen mixes with our blood, and it is carried to every cell, fiber, and organ in the body; when we exhale, carbon dioxide is released. The more oxygen that we have in our blood, the healthier our bodies are. When air is not properly expelled by breathing properly, our system is poisoned by waste products or toxins that are not eliminated in the blood. In our modern, stressed world most people breathe incorrectly with shallow breaths that only exercise the tops of the lungs. By practicing pranayama exercises we expand our capacity to take in oxygen by up to seven times the average amount. This helps to activate the body's circulatory system, promoting a healthy appetite, proper digestion, and encouraging sound sleep.

THE BENEFITS OF PRACTICE

If practiced properly, pranayama purifies the nervous system and concentrates the mind in preparation for the higher stages of yoga, namely meditation. Because breathing exercises activate the major organs of the body —the heart, lungs and brain—and benefit the nervous system, they should never be practiced without an experienced teacher. The exercises given here are preparatory exercises for advanced pranayama techniques.

Never practice breathing exercises in a hurry or force them. The four important aspects of the breath are inhalation, exhalation, internal breath retention, and external breath retention, which will be utilized in all the breathing exercises that are given here.

nadi suddhi

Nerve purification breath

Practice this breathing exercise before Meditation (see p.113)

1 Sit on the floor in a comfortable meditation posture with your spine erect. Bend your right arm and take your right hand into *vishnu* mudra by bending your fore and index fingers. Relax your face.

2 Close your right nostril with the thumb of your right hand. **Inhale,** then as you **exhale:** completely breathe out all the air from your lungs through your left nostril without straining. **Inhale:** slowly and deeply inhale through the same nostril to the count of four, then **exhale.** Expand your stomach muscles as you inhale to pull in more air.

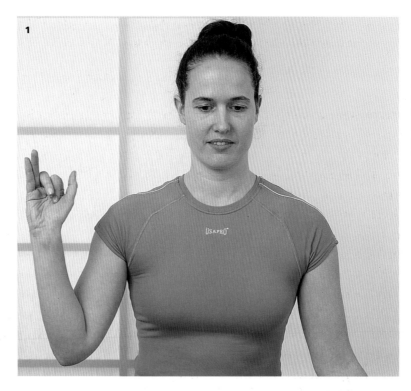

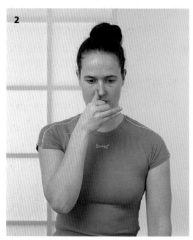

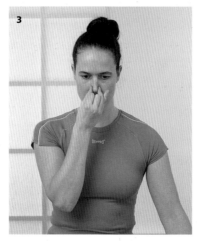

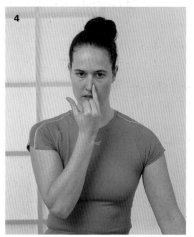

3 Close both nostrils with your thumb and fingers, holding your left nostril down with your ring and little fingers.
Breath: hold your breath internally to the count of eight, without straining.

4 **Exhale:** let go with your thumb and release your breath. as you let go of your right nostril.
Inhale then as you **exhale:** breathe out very slowly to the count of eight, so your exhalation is twice as long as the inhalation.
Inhale: breathe in to the count of four through the same nostril.
Exhale: close both nostrils and repeat cycle at least ten times. Release nostrils and breathe normally.

kapalabhati

Shining skull breath

This rapid diaphragmatic breathing removes carbon dioxide and impurities from the body and helps to clear the sinuses and lungs.

Inhale, then quickly contract the abdomen to **exhale:** relax the abdomen and air will automatically be drawn into the lungs. Follow these two movements in quick succession. Do 3–5 rounds of this exercise, allowing 20–30 contractions each time. **Breath:** release and take a deep breath in, followed by an extended exhalation. Then return to normal breathing. If you feel dizzy while practicing kapalabhati, then stop or slow down the contractions of the abdomen.

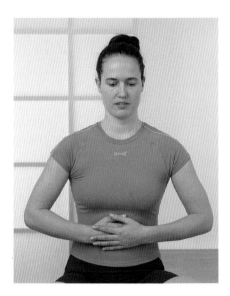

deergha swaasam

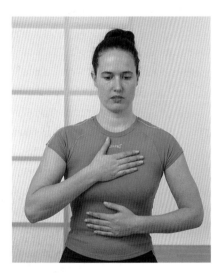

Full yogic breath

Breathing comprises a three-step process.
Inhale: firstly, breathe in by expanding your abdomen, drawing air to your lower lungs. Then expand your ribcage, taking air into the middle of your lungs, then finally lift your collarbones to bring air to the top of your lungs. Hold briefly.
Exhale: breathe out in reverse order, releasing it from the upper, middle and lower lungs. Then employ external breath retention (see above) for a few seconds before you inhale again. Make both the inhalation and exhalation one continuous flow. Repeat 3–5 times, then return to normal breathing.

ujjayi breathing

Victorious breath while lying

Sit cross-legged in *sukhasana* (see p.114) then lie back on a bolster, so that your ribs are supported and your spine is on the center of the bolster. Relax your arms out to the sides, palms up, and let your shoulders drop down. Tuck your chin in slightly to extend the back of your neck, and relax your face. Gently contract your glottis to produce a soft snoring sound at the back of the throat as you breathe.
Inhale: breathe in slowly and deeply.
Exhale: breathe out, slowly emptying your lungs without straining.

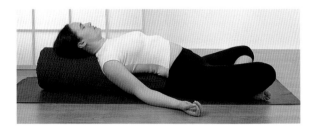

Breath: your breathing should be soft, elongated and rhythmic like the sound of the ocean. A simultaneous contraction of the abdomen should happen automatically as you breathe.

Meditation

There are many benefits to meditation. By sitting still and concentrating the mind, you slow your heart rate and breathing, which greatly reduces stress. Meditation has also been shown to decrease the rate at which cells decay, therefore slowing the aging process. People who meditate regularly seem to remain buoyant throughout the ups and downs of life.

PREPARING TO MEDITATE

Meditate in a quiet area in your home, preferably the same location and same time daily—early morning is good. This is because developing a regular habit is essential to gaining mastery of the mind. Meditate for 20 minutes daily, then slowly increase to one hour.

THE BEST WAY TO SIT

To keep your mind steady and focused, a comfortable posture is needed. Sit in any of the poses detailed in this section. You can also sit on a dining chair with a straight spine. If you sit on the floor, place a cushion under your buttocks to raise your hips and prevent any back strain. Sit straight with your shoulders level, keeping your head in line with your spine (see right). Your body should be at ease. Also relax your face. Half close your eyes, and start to mentally bring your gaze inward.

Breath links your body and your mind, so breathe evenly. Try not to move when meditating. If you have any discomfort, make a minor adjustment, but avoid fidgeting. Also do not allow yourself to fall asleep.

HOW TO MEDITATE

Different techniques can focus your mind to begin meditation. Some people use a home altar. To prepare one, cover a small table with an attractive cloth. Place an inspirational image on it, such as a statue of Buddha or a deity. You can add a candle, flowers, or a yantra (a mystical symbol or geometric diagram), as they are all useful meditation tools. Incense can relax you and help still your mind.

To meditate using an object such as a lit candle, first concentrate on the object and simply observe the flame. Avoid being distracted by any thoughts that arise in your mind about the object. Then close your eyes and see the flame; repeat the exercise.

Meditating with a mantra is also useful. Mantras are sacred sounds heard by ancient sages while meditating. The sounds are believed to set off sympathetic vibrations within the body that tune it into higher frequencies. Common mantras include *OM* or *OM Shanti*.

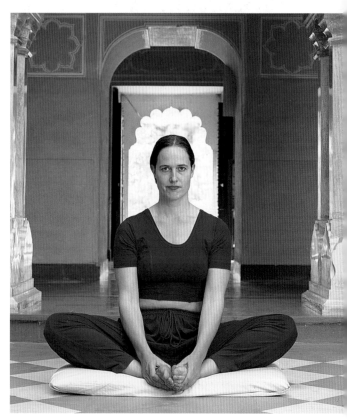

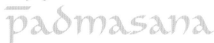

padmasana

Lotus

This is a classic sitting pose ideal for meditation for someone advanced in yoga practice.

Sit upright in *dandasana* pose (see p.56). Bend your right leg. Take hold of your right foot at the ankle with both hands, and place your foot on top of your left thigh with the sole facing up. Bend your left leg and holding your left foot lift it onto your right thigh. Keep your body straight with hips, shoulders, and head in line. Place your hands, palms up, on your knees.

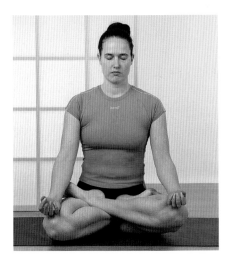

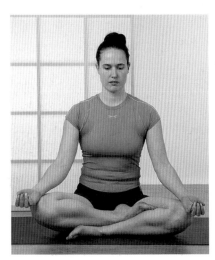

ardha padmasana

Half lotus

An intermediate cross-legged pose that is comfortable for meditation and begins to open the hips in preparation for full lotus pose.

Sit upright in *dandasana* pose (see p.56). Bend your left leg and holding your left foot place the heel close to your right groin, sole facing up. Bend your right leg and place your right foot on your left calf. Sit straight with your hands, palms facing upward, on your knees.

sukhasana

Happy pose

A simple meditation pose for beginners, or people suffering from knee problems.

Sit upright in *dandasana* pose (see p.56). Bend both legs, crossing your right shin over your left. Sit straight with your hips, shoulders, and head in line. Place your hands on the tops of your knees with your palms facing upward.

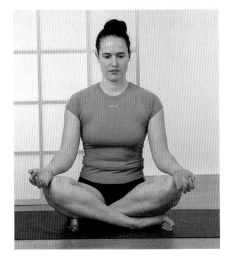

vīrasana

Hero pose

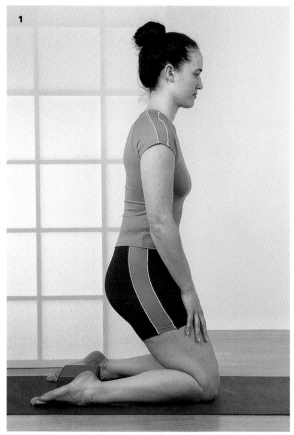

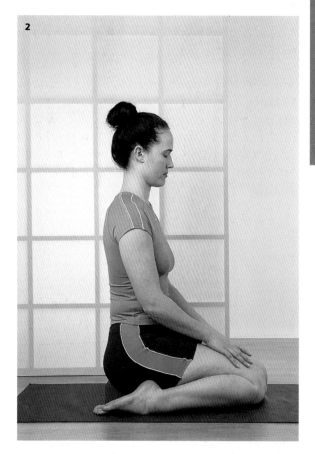

This is a kneeling pose that keeps the spine erect for meditation and is useful for people who suffer from tight hips.

1 From a kneeling position, lift up your buttocks so that you are balancing on your knees. Keep your knees together and move your feet a little wider than a hip-width apart, with your toes pointing backward. Rest your hands on your thighs.

2 Slowly sit back down between your feet, easing your calf muscles out to the sides with your thumbs as you sit back (see *triang mukhaikapada paschimottanasana* pp.60–61). Sit up straight lifting up from the sit bones in your buttocks. Place your hands on top of your knees. Put a folded blanket or cushion under your sit bones, so that you are more comfortable in the pose during meditation.

Workouts

Practice becomes firmly grounded when well attended to for a long time, without a break and in all earnestness.

The yoga sutra of Patanjali 1:14

As is written in the first chapter of the yoga sutra, in order to experience the fruits of yoga it has to be practiced consistently. Practice for a short period every day, rather than doing a long exhausting session once a week. If you cannot practice daily, then try to do one of the workouts detailed at least twice a week. It will take at least three months before you will notice any changes.

WHEN TO PRACTICE

Practice yoga at home either in the early morning, when the mind is clear but the body is stiff, or early evening when the body is warmed up but the mind is over-active. Find a warm, clear area that is large enough for a sticky yoga mat. Woman should not practice any inversions during the first two days of menstruation, or after the fourth month of pregnancy.

This section offers five basic workouts: a 30-minute program; an easy yoga workout for beginners; a more challenging practice for intermediate and advanced students; an energizing workout; a de-stressing workout; plus a safe yoga program for people with back pain. Do the poses once; repeat only if a number is shown in brackets.

The short 30-minute workout, opposite, can be practiced daily, and is ideal for busy people as it can be easily fitted into the daily routine.

30-minute yoga workout

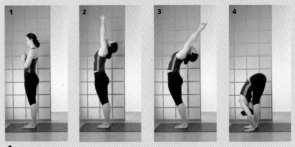

1 *Surya namaskar/Sun salutation pp.32–35*

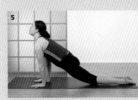 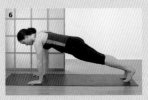

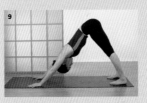 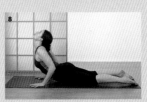

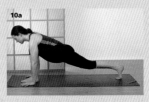

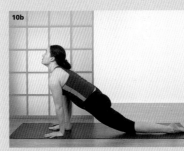 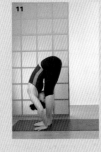

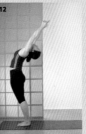 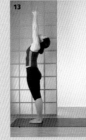 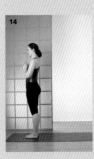

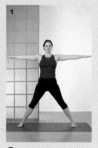 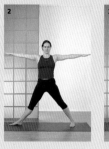 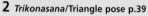 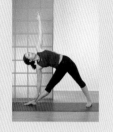 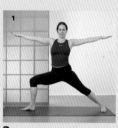 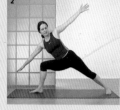

2 *Trikonasana*/Triangle pose p.39   **3** *Parsvakonasana*/Extended side stretch p.41

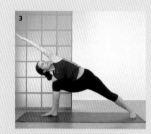 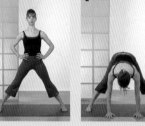 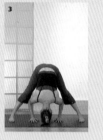 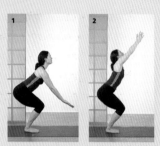

4 *Padottanasana*/Extended leg pose p.43   **5** *Utkatasana*/Powerful pose p.51

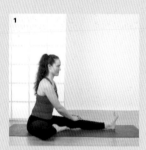 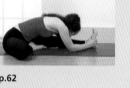 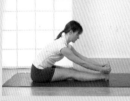 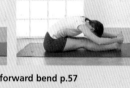

6 *Janu sirsasana*/Head to knee pose p.62   **7** *Paschimottanasana*/Seated forward bend p.57

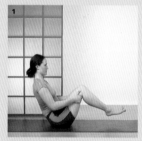 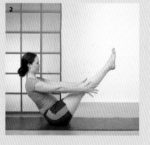 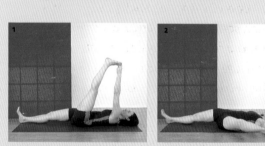

8 *Navasana*/Boat pose p.80   **9** *Supta padangusthasana*/Lying thumb to foot pose p.86

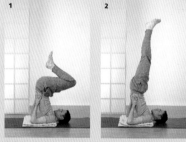 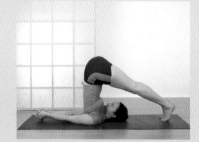 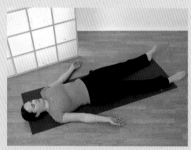

10 *Sarvangasana*/Shoulder stand p.104   **11** Shoulder stand with both legs down p.106   **12** *Savasana*/Relaxation pose p.107

Easy yoga workout—1 hr

For beginners to yoga, it is important to attend a class to get some basic instruction, but this easy workout can be practiced between classes. Do not force your body to perfect a pose. Rather, do a posture to the best of your ability, keep breathing steadily throughout, and simply observe the areas of your body that are feeling tight.

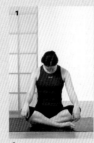 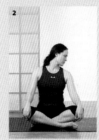 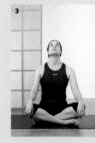 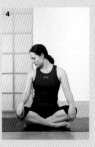

1 Head rolls p.22

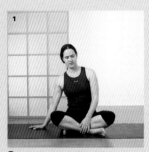 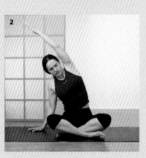 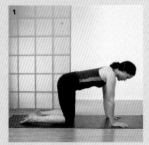 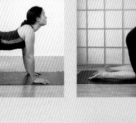

2 Sitting side stretch p.23

3 Sitting forward stretch p.24

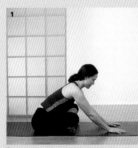 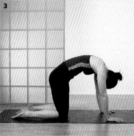 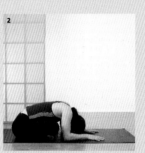

4 Cat stretch p.30

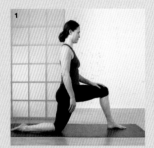 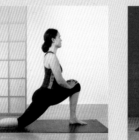 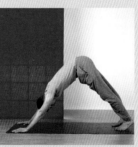

5 Lunge p.31

6 *Adho mukha svanasana*/Downward facing dog p.89

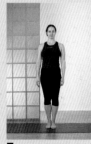 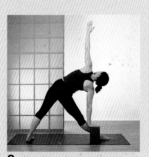 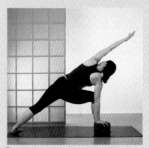

7 *Tadasana*/Mountain pose p.38

8 *Trikonasana*/Triangle pose, beginner's version p.39

9 *Parsvakonasana*/Extended side stretch, beginner's version p.41

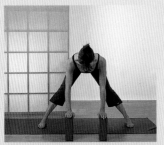

10 *Padottanasana*/Extended leg pose
– beginner's version p.43

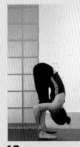

11 *Vrksasana*/Tree pose p.50

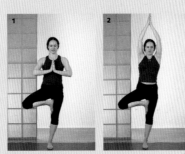

12 *Uttanasana*/Standing forward bend p.53

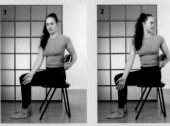

13 *Bharadvajasana*/Twisting on a chair p.74

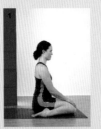

14 *Supta virasana*/
Hero pose, Step 1 p.88

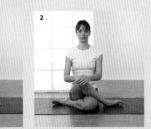

15 *Gomukasana*/Cow face pose pp.66–67

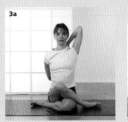

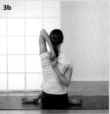

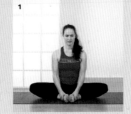

16 *Baddha konasana*/Cobbler pose
Step 1 p.69

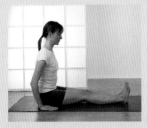

17 *Dandasana*/Staff pose p.56

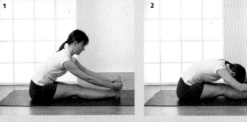

18 *Paschimottanasana*/Seated forward bend p.57

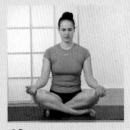

19 *Sukhasana*/Happy pose
p.114

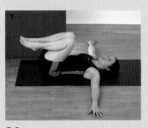

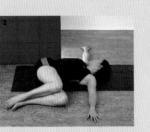

20 *Parivartanasana*/Lying side stretch p.87

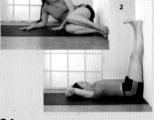

21 *Viparita karani*/Legs up the wall
p.107

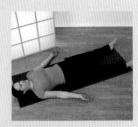

22 *Savasana*/Relaxation
pose p.107

Intermediate/advanced yoga workout—1 hr 15 min

This more challenging workout emphasizes concentration and balance in the poses. You should practice this workout only if you have been doing yoga for two years and can hold *Sirsasana* (headstand) for 5 minutes.

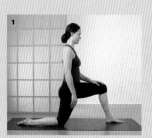
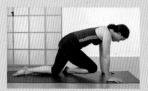
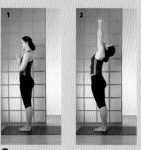

1 Buttock stretch p.25

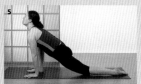
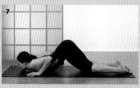

2 Lunge p.31

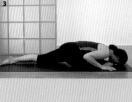
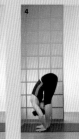
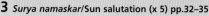
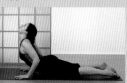

3 *Surya namaskar*/Sun salutation (x 5) pp.32–35

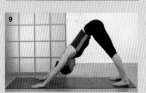
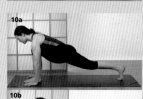
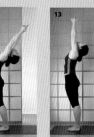
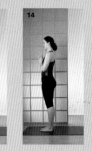

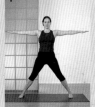
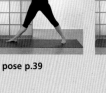
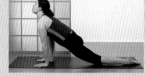
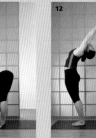
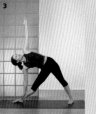

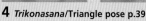

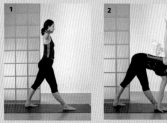

4 *Trikonasana*/Triangle pose p.39

5 *Parivrtta trikonasana*/Reverse triangle pose p.40

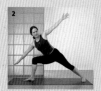
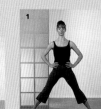
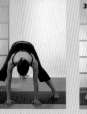

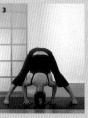
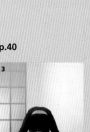

6 *Parsvakonasana*/Extended side stretch p.41

7 *Padottanasana*/Extended leg pose p.43

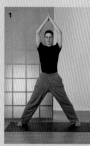 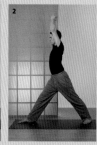 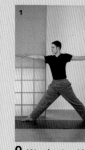 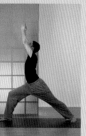 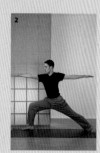

8 *Virabhadrasana*/Warrior p.48   **9** Warrior I p.49

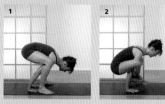 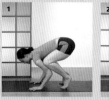 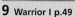 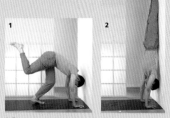

10 *Bhujapidasana*/Arm pressure pose p.81   **11** *Bakasana*/Crow p.82   **12** *Adho mukha vrksasana*/Face down tree pose p.98

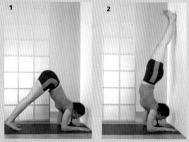 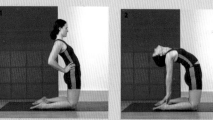

13 *Pinca mayurasana*/Peacock pose p.99   **14** *Ustrasana*/Camel pose p.93

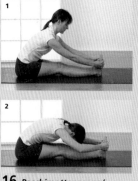

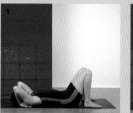 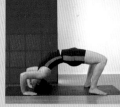 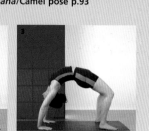

15 *Urdhva dhanurasana*/Upward bow pose (x 3) p.95   **16** *Paschimottanasana*/Seated forward bend p.57

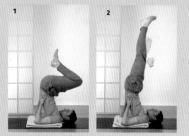 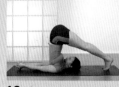 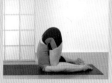 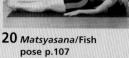

17 *Sarvangasana*/Shoulder stand p.104   **18** Shoulder stand with knees by ears p.106   **19** Shoulder stand with both legs down p.106   **20** *Matsyasana*/Fish pose p.107

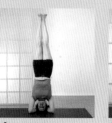 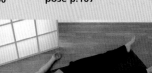 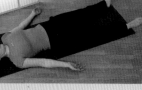

21 *Sirsasana*/Headstand p.102   **22** *Padmasana*/Lotus p.114   **23** *Savasana*/Relaxation pose p.107

Energizing yoga workout—1 hr 15 min

Practicing this energizing workout regularly will give a real boost to a sluggish body. Beginners to yoga should omit the headstand and the upward bow, and intermediate practitioners should include a headstand only if they are confident that they can practice it well on their own.

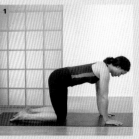

1 Cat stretch p.30

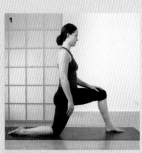

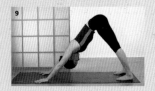 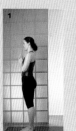 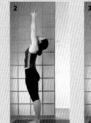

2 Lunge p.31

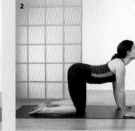 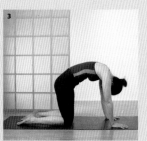

3 Arm circles p.29

4 *Surya namaskar*/Sun salutation (x5) pp.32–35

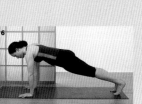

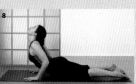

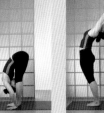 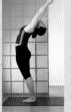 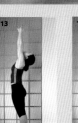 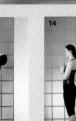 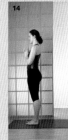 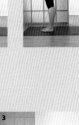

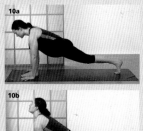 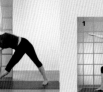 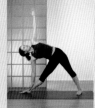

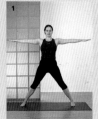 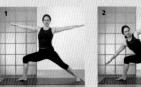 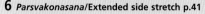

5 *Trikonasana*/Triangle pose p.39   **6** *Parsvakonasana*/Extended side stretch p.41

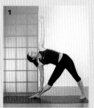 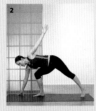 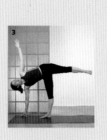

7 *Ardha chandrasana*/Half moon pose p.44

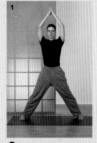 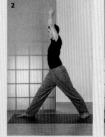

8 *Virabhadrasana*/Warrior pose p.48

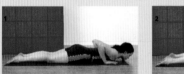 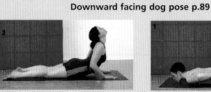 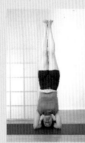

9 Warrior I pose p.49

10 *Adho mukha svanasana*/
Downward facing dog pose p.89

11 *Sirsasana*/Headstand p.102

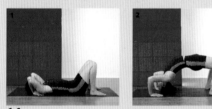 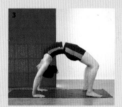 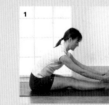 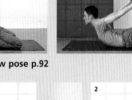

12 *Bhujangasana*/Cobra pose p.90

13 *Dhanurasana*/Bow pose p.92

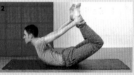 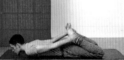 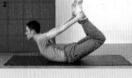

14 *Urdhva dhanurasana*/Upward bow pose (x 3) p.95

15 *Paschimottanasana*/Seated forward bend p.57

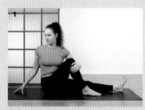 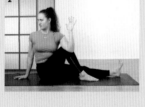 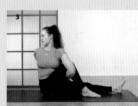 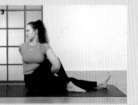 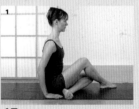

16 *Marichyasana III* p.76

17 *Ardha matsyendrasana* p.75

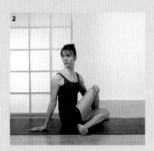 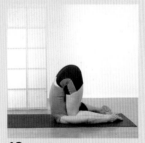 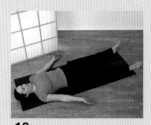

18 Shoulder stand with knees by ears p.106

19 *Savasana*/Relaxation pose p.107

123

De-stressing yoga workout—1 hr 15 min

This is a good workout to do if you have a stressful job or lifestyle, as it will help to calm your mind and balance your emotions.

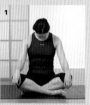
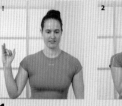
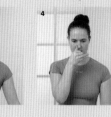
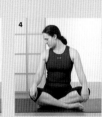
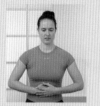

1 *Nadi suddhi*/Nerve purification breath p.111

2 *Kapalabhati*/Shining skull breath p.112

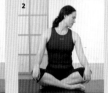
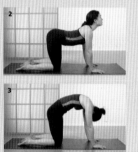
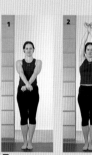
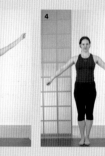

3 Head rolls p.22

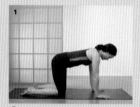
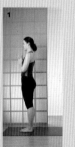
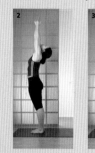
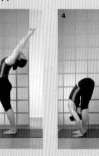

4 Cat stretch p.30

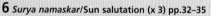

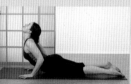
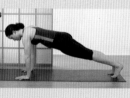
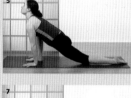
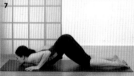

5 Arm circles p.29

6 *Surya namaskar*/Sun salutation (x 3) pp.32–35

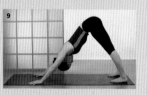
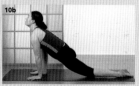
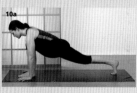
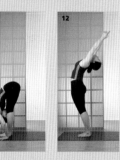
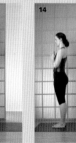
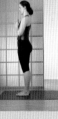

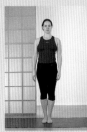

7 *Tadasana*/Mountain pose p.38

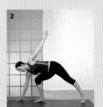

8 *Uttanasana*/Forward bend p.53

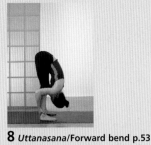

9 *Trikonasana*/Triangle pose p.39

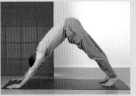

10 *Ardha chandrasana*/Half moon pose p.44

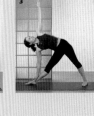

11 *Padottanasana*/Extended leg pose p.43

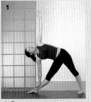

12 *Adho mukha svanasana*/ Downward facing dog pose p.89

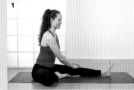
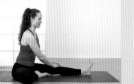

13 *Janu sirsasana*/Head to knee pose p.62

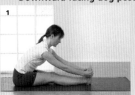

14 *Paschimottanasana*/Seated forward bend p.57

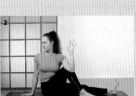
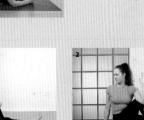

15 *Marichyasana III* p.76

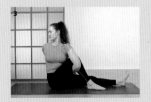
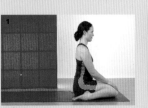

16 *Supta virasana*/Hero pose p.88

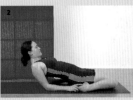
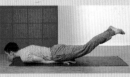

17 *Bhujangasana*/Cobra pose p.90

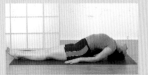

18 *Salabhasana*/Locust pose p.91

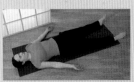

19 Child's pose p.101

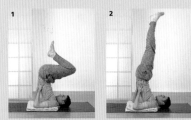

20 *Sarvangasana*/Shoulder stand p.104

21 Shoulder stand with knees by ears p.106

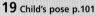

22 *Matsyasana*/Fish pose p.107

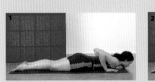

23 *Savasana*/Relaxation pose p.107

Yoga for bad backs workout—45 min

This is a gentle workout to release tension and stiffness in the back. If you are experiencing back pain, approach all the exercises with caution and do not rush them. Practice the pose to the edge of your pain and then release it. Do not continue with any pose if it aggravates your discomfort.

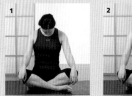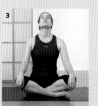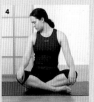

1 Head rolls p.22

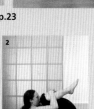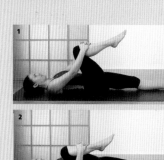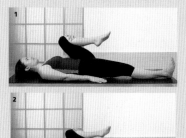

2 Sitting side stretch p.23

3 One knee to chest p.26

4 One knee to the side p.27

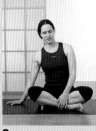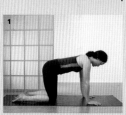

5 Head to knees p.28

6 Cat stretch p.30

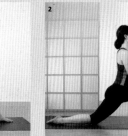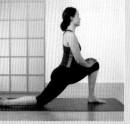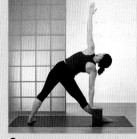

7 Lunge p.31

8 *Tadasana*/Mountain pose p.38

9 *Trikonasana*/Triangle pose, beginner's version p.39

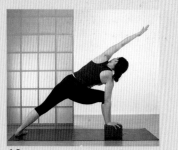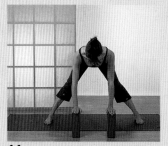

10 *Parsvakonasana*/Extended side stretch, beginner's version p.41

11 *Padottanasana*/Extended leg pose, beginner's version p.43

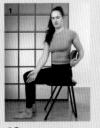 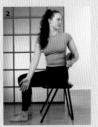 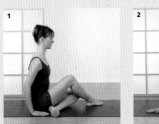 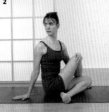 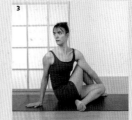

12 *Bharadvajasana*/Twisting on a chair p.74 **13** *Ardha matsyendrasana* p.75

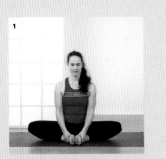 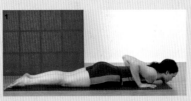 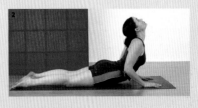

14 *Baddha konasana*/Cobbler pose Step 1 p.69 **15** *Bhujangasana*/Cobra pose (x 3) p.90

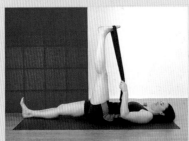 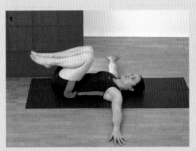 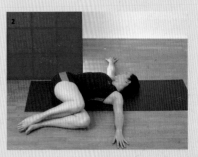

16 *Supta padangusthasana*/Lying thumb to foot pose, beginner's version p.86 **17** *Parivartanasana*/Lying side stretch p.87

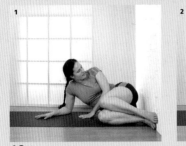 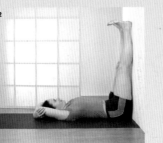 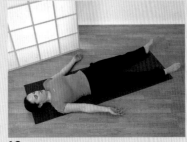 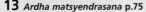

18 *Viparita karani*/Legs up the wall p.107 **19** *Savasana*/Relaxation pose p.107

Index